Art Therapy for Groups

Art Therapy for Groups is a valuable introduction to art therapy and groupwork. It explains the reasons for using theme-based groupwork and provides detailed guidance on how to set up and run a theme-based art therapy group. All aspects of the therapy are considered – equal opportunities, size of groups, common problems, safety – across a broad range of groups, from residential institutions to community situations.

This new edition presents nearly 400 themes and practical exercises to use with groups, set out in sections ranging from personal work to group interactive exercises. Fresh material includes:

- Consideration of race, culture, diversity and equal opportunity
- A chapter on recording, evaluation and evidence-based practice
- A survey of literature on art therapy groups, leading to a summary of models used in art therapy with groups
- Seventy new themes collected from art therapists' responses
- An updated international resources section acknowledging a more global outlook

Illustrated by more new black and white photographs this book is an essential resource for all people working with art therapy and personal art groups.

Marian Liebmann has worked as a teacher, community worker, probation officer and art therapist. She has work in art therapy with offenders, with women's groups and community groups, and currently at the Inner City Mental Health Service in Bristol. She teaches and lectures on art therapy at several universities in the UK and Ireland. She also works in mediation and conflict resolution, and has run Art and Conflict workshops in many countries. She has written and edited seven books on art therapy and mediation, and many chapters in other books.

Art Therapy for Groups

A handbook of themes and exercises

Second Edition

Marian Liebmann

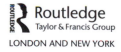
Routledge
Taylor & Francis Group
LONDON AND NEW YORK

First edition published 1986 by Croom Helm Ltd and Brookline Books
Reprinted 1987

Reprinted 1989, 1991, 1994, 1997, 1999 by Routledge

Reprinted 2001 by Routledge

Second edition published 2004 by Routledge
27 Church Road, Hove, East Sussex BN3 2FA

Simultaneously published in the USA and Canada
Routledge
290 Madison Avenue, New York NY 10016

Reprinted 2005 (twice) and 2007

Routledge is an imprint of the Taylor & Francis Group, an Informa business

Copyright © 2004 Mary Liebmann

Typeset in Times by Mayhew Typesetting, Rhayader, Powys
Printed and bound in Great Britain by Biddles Ltd, King's Lynn, Norfolk
Cover design by Jim Wilkie

This publication has been produced with paper manufactured to strict
environmental standards and with pulp derived from sustainable
forests.

British Library Cataloguing in Publication Data
A catalogue record for this book is available from the British Library

Library of Congress Cataloguing in Publication Data
Liebmann, Marian, 1942–
  Art therapy for groups : a handbook of themes and exercises /
Marian Liebmann – 2nd ed.
        p. : cm.
Includes bibliographical references and indexes.
  ISBN 1-58391-217-7 (hbk.) – ISBN 1-58391-218-5 (pbk.)
  1. Art therapy–Handbooks, manuals, etc. 2. Group
psychotherapy–Handbooks, manuals, etc.
  [DNLM: 1. Art therapy–methods. 2. Psychotherapy, Group–
methods.
WM 450.5.A8 L716a 2004] I. Title.

  RC489.A7L54 2004
  616.89′1656–dc22

                                                      2003017297

ISBN 978-1-58391-218-8

Contents

Figures

In the list below, photographers' names appear in brackets. The photographs are not all to the same scale.

Line drawings for heading sections in Part II are by the author

Acknowledgements to first edition

This book has drawn on the experiences of many people.

First, I would like to thank my tutor, Michael Edwards, who helped me ask the right questions for my dissertation, which was the forerunner of this book. Next, my thanks go to all the art therapists and others who trusted me with their ideas; their names are listed at the back of the book.

Members of Bristol Art Therapy Group have been a great support to me, in encouraging me to produce the original collection, in talking to me about their work and in constructively criticising the manuscript of the present version of the book. Special thanks to Sheena Anderson, Heather Buddery, Paul Curtis, Michael Donnelly, Karen Lee Drucker, John Ford, Linnea Lowes and Roy Thornton.

The participants of the 'Friday Group' (Bristol Art and Psychology Group) took a great interest in the progress of the book in its formative stages. Patricia Brownen and Beryl Tyzack read the whole manuscript and others commented on small sections.

Experts from other fields helped with booklists: Allan Brown on group-work, Sue Jennings on dramatherapy, Alison Levinge on music therapy. Sue Jennings also advised on the manuscript, as did my friend June Boyce-Tillman who is also a writer.

Finally, my thanks to my husband, Mike Coldham, who helped by checking the readability and coherence of the text, as well as providing much practical support; and to my daughter, Anna, for her considerable patience.

Marian Liebmann
1986

Acknowledgements to second edition

I am extremely grateful for the help and support of a great many people. Without this help, the second edition could not have been produced. Like the African proverb 'It takes a village to raise a child', it takes a community to produce a book of this kind.

My community of art therapists in Bristol helped by acting as a sounding board for ideas and reading and commenting on most of the new material. I would particularly like to thank Nadija Corcos, Karen Lee Drucker, Nicky Linfield and Liz Lumley-Smith.

The Art Therapy, Race and Culture (ARC) Group of the British Association of Art Therapists helped with suggesting ideas, advising on equal opportunity and cultural issues, and reading several chapters. I would like to thank Frederica Brooks, Jean Campbell and Cathy Ward in this respect.

I would like to thank Dorothy Stock Whitaker for her helpful and detailed comments on the proposal and the chapters, especially concerning groupwork.

Many people helped with Chapter 3, which is entirely new. In addition to the people above, my thanks go to Andrea Gilroy, Val Huet, Kevin Jones, Rosie Jones, Sarah Lewis, Richard Manners, John Mellor-Clark, Susan Rooke-Matthews, Kate Rothwell and Tony Soteriou. Between them they encompass art therapy, psychology, research and development, and service user perspectives.

Those who contributed new themes and exercises, and those who helped with lists of books and organisations are in the List of Contributors, which can be found on pp. 321–2.

In addition are those who gave me information or put me in contact with relevant people or resources, too numerous to mention. And if I have forgotten anyone, please forgive me!

Last, but not least, my thanks to my husband, Mike Coldham, for his patience and never-ending supply of meals and practical help during the whole process.

Marian Liebmann
2004

Preface to first edition

The starting point of this book was my own experience as a member of several groups and the leader of others. I had always been interested in art and became more and more interested in its potential for the communication of personal matters. I became a staff member at an experimental day centre for adult ex-offenders and ran sessions there. I also ran day events for church groups and the local encounter centre. At the same time I attended any group art sessions within reach to gain more personal experience. I began to compile a list of games, structures, themes – call them what you will – that other group leaders used and added them to those that I or my groups invented. I also became very curious about groups and the structures they used, and how these influenced what went on in the groups.

I decided to pursue this interest further and in 1979 I enrolled for the MA course in art therapy at Birmingham Polytechnic. For my dissertation I chose to explore my interest in structured art therapy groups and devised a questionnaire to use as a basis to interview 40 art therapists working in different settings; not all of them were officially called 'art therapists' but they were all using art as a means of personal communication. It was a fascinating learning experience for me and some of my findings are included in Chapter 1.

One of the purposes I had in mind was to produce a collection of all the themes being used by art therapists, teachers and group leaders. This had to be done after the dissertation as there was simply too much material to include. With the help of other art therapists in Bristol, the collection was produced in 1982 as a handbook to circulate to those who took part in my survey and other interested art therapists.

This handbook assumed its readers would all be art therapists experienced in running groups, so it contained no material on this aspect. However, since its publication, there has been widespread interest shown by occupational therapists, social workers, teachers, child guidance workers, community group leaders, peace activists and others. This burgeoning interest shows a need for a new version with more material on how to run groups and ways in which themes may be used with different groups. These topics form the first half of the book, and the updated collection of themes forms the second half.

Marian Liebmann
1986

Preface to second edition

When the first edition of this book was published in 1986, it was the second book on art therapy to be published in the UK. During the years that have elapsed since then, this situation has changed dramatically and there are now many books on art therapy, including several on working with groups. Art therapy has become much more established in an ever-widening range of settings. My own art therapy practice has deepened and taken on other perspectives. However, there still seems to be a place for this book, which has become popular in many quarters, as witnessed by editions in Hebrew, Portuguese and Chinese.

When Brunner-Routledge asked if I was interested in producing a new edition, I could think immediately of many things which needed updating: our client language has changed; the concept of 'games' is no longer used much; the book needed a 'race, culture, diversity and equal opportunity' perspective. But I also needed to find out from others what was missing and what might better be omitted.

As preparation for the second edition, I carried out a survey of some of those who have used the book. I advertised in the British Association of Art Therapists (BAAT) newsletter and also among local art therapists. I sent out 21 questionnaires and received 12 responses. I also talked to many art therapists and to the Art Therapy, Race and Culture (ARC) group of the British Association of Art Therapists. All their suggestions helped me formulate more precisely the changes needed. It has taken three years to compile the second edition and as it neared completion it became clear that a chapter on evaluation and evidence-based practice was needed. The main changes to the book are:

- a complete overhaul of the language and terminology towards a less stigmatising view of clients
- a race, culture, diversity and equal opportunity perspective: rather than introduce a new section for this, I have tried to ensure that it is incorporated throughout the text

- a survey of literature on art therapy groups, leading to a summary of models used in art therapy with groups
- more detail on some aspects of running a group, including greater attention to safety factors
- a new chapter on recording, evaluation and evidence-based practice
- eight new accounts of examples of groups, including three looking at race and culture issues
- about 70 new themes and many new variations on existing ones, collected mainly from art therapists' responses
- a completely new Resources section, including up-to-date books and an international set of addresses to acknowledge a more global outlook.

I hope this second edition of the book will continue to serve many people, as the first one has done.

Marian Liebmann
2004

Introduction

Who this book is for

This book is aimed primarily at professionals in a wide variety of caring professions who are interested in developing their skills and experience in using art with groups. They may be art therapists, teachers, social workers, youth workers or community group leaders. This book will also be of interest to group therapists, managers of therapeutic services and teachers providing courses for the caring professions.

Understanding and facilitating an art therapy group requires knowledge of groups and how they function and develop, and skills in using art in this context. This book assumes knowledge and experience of working with groups and concentrates on how to use art with groups. However, if you do not have much experience in running groups, there is a list of books on groupwork in the bibliography at the end of the book. There are also many courses now available on groupwork of different kinds. But there is no substitute for experience and the only way to gain this is to join a variety of groups as a client or member. This gives you an opportunity both to experience what it feels like to be in the client role and to observe different styles of facilitating groups.

Then you will need to co-facilitate some groups with an experienced facilitator or therapist. This gives you a chance to learn from someone more experienced, to try out your ideas and skills gradually, and to discuss the results. When you feel ready to facilitate your own groups, it is a good practice to work with a colleague and also to obtain supervision from another experienced person not involved with your group.

The same goes for experience of using art. It can be a powerful experience, so it is essential to know what it feels like. Sometimes it is difficult to get started or to make something as you envisaged it. If you have not experienced this yourself you will not be able to help others when they are stuck. A helpful guideline is always to try out on yourself and your colleagues what you are intending to use with clients. This experience may give you pointers about possible difficulties, iron out organisational wrinkles and demonstrate benefits which can be gained.

The people running the group may be called therapists, facilitators, leaders, teachers, social workers, group workers, etc. depending on the setting. People attending groups may be called patients, clients, participants, members or just 'people'. I will use therapist or facilitator for the person(s) running the group, and whatever term seems appropriate in the context for the participants.

Qualified art therapists may be able to help. They have all undertaken specialist training in this field. The British Association of Art Therapists (address in Resources section at end of book) can put you in touch with the regional group contact in your area for advice.

Groups and individuals

Although this book has been written with groups in mind, many of the themes in Part II can be used in working with individuals, except for those exercises which require pairs or groups. It is important to make some arrangement for individuals to share their work with someone and to discuss any feelings arising from it.

There are many places (such as day centres and hospitals) where an art therapy or personal art group may be part of a larger programme, including individual counselling, other therapy groups, community meetings, etc. In such contexts staff liaison is very important. This book applies to these situations as much as 'stand-alone' groups.

Ways of using this book

If you are new to this kind of work, it will pay dividends to read the whole of Part I. Then, assuming you have some experience of groups, think about the group you are working with and think about members' individual needs. Pick a relevant exercise and try it out on yourself and your colleagues. After that, introduce it (perhaps with modifications) to your group. The results of that will determine what follows (see Chapter 2 for more details of how to choose themes).

If you are already familiar with running this kind of group, a good way of using this book is to browse through it and let it trigger off your own thoughts. You can then choose an exercise and modify it to suit your particular situation, or make up your own entirely.

What this book does and does not cover

1   This book covers groups which meet to share a common activity or theme and does not cover groups where everyone chooses a different activity.

2   This book is an attempt to provide an ordered framework around what is essentially an intuitive process. To use a metaphor, a book on sailing can outline the equipment needed before you start, provide a chart of where dangerous currents might be and give a few accounts of actual sailing trips. It is then up to you to set sail and see what sailing is really like.

3   Not all themes are for everyone. Never use an exercise or theme you feel unhappy with yourself.

4   This book does not make novices into instant therapists or facilitators. Training and experience, both as a client and as co-facilitator, are most important.

5   A personal art group will not necessarily change people's lives (though it can) – many factors are involved.

6   This book has no guidance about long-term therapeutic work. If you intend to work in this area, make sure you have the necessary qualifications, expertise, support and supervision.

7   This book contains examples of art therapy groups drawn from many client groups, but does not cover specific characteristics of different client groups in detail.

8   Experience of what is involved in painting or making something is a very important part of this work.

Race, culture, diversity and equality issues

With the advent of the Race Relations Amendment Act (2000), implemented from 31 May 2002, all public authorities have a statutory duty to promote race equality. The aim is to help public authorities to provide fair and accessible services, and to make the promotion of race equality central to their work. Public authorities are expected to take the lead in promoting equality of opportunity and good race relations, and in preventing unlawful discrimination. This means that they must take account of race equality in policies and service delivery (Commission for Racial Equality 2003).

The first edition of this book paid no attention to race, culture or diversity issues – they were just not within many professionals' consciousness as areas of reflection and practice. Racism and discrimination have, of course, existed from time immemorial, but it is only fairly recently that we have realised our obligations and abilities to do something about them, wherever we are. Cultural issues too have always been present, but we are now increasingly trying to work with difference in a positive way.

Diversity includes a wide range of issues: race, culture, disability, class, gender, age, religion, health – in fact any area where people may be discriminated against through being labelled as part of a group; e.g. being refused services because of living on a certain housing estate. As well as striving to provide a service for all people equally, agencies and organisations are learning more creative ways of working with difference. This is all part of providing effective services that meet all communities' needs and doing so in a professional way. Throughout this book I will try to pay attention to these issues in such a way as to make this a resource which is inclusive and helps to celebrate our diversity.

References

Commission for Racial Equality (CRE) (2003) 'The duty to promote race equality'. Online: www.cre.gov.uk/duty/index.html (accessed 6 January 2003).

PART I

Art therapy groups

Chapter 1

Art therapy and groupwork

This chapter gives some definitions of art therapy and a brief outline of its historical development. It lists several of the benefits of art therapy, including its value with diversity issues, and discusses the overlaps between art therapy and art activities. It looks at the reasons for using groups. It goes on to give some background to personal art and art therapy groups, drawing on a survey of 40 art therapists and group facilitators running art/art therapy groups in a variety of settings, and identifies therapeutic factors in groups. The emergence of several models of art therapy groupwork is charted. Reasons for using themes are noted and the chapter finishes with a look at the flexible use of themes.

Art therapy: some definitions

Art therapy uses art as a means of personal expression to communicate feelings, rather than aiming at aesthetically pleasing end products to be judged by external standards. This means of expression is available to everyone, not just the artistically gifted. There are many definitions of art therapy – here is one based on working in a therapy setting:

> Art therapy involves the use of different art media through which a patient can express and work through the issues and concerns that have brought him or her into therapy. The therapist and client are in partnership in trying to understand the art process and product of the session.
>
> (Case and Dalley 1992: 1)

Here is a wider definition including all arts therapies and other settings:

> The common ground for all arts therapies includes the focus on non-verbal communication and creative processes together with the facilitation of a trusting, safe environment within which people can acknowledge and express strong emotions.
>
> (Payne 1993: xi)

As will be seen from the examples given further on in Chapter 6, art therapy can be relevant to many people, whether they are grappling with serious problems or just wish to explore themselves and their feelings, using art as the medium. In the words of one art therapist, running a group for the general public: 'No special ability or disability is required.'

Art therapy: a brief history

The history of art therapy derives from several different strands. The first is from work done in child art. Franz Cizek, a progressive art educator in Austria around 1900, believed in children having 'free expression' in art, and arranged an exhibition of child art in 1908. As his ideas spread, he brought the exhibition to London in 1934–5. In England, Marion Richardson promoted the idea and spontaneous work in children's art classes became widespread during the 1940s (Waller 1991).

A second strand arose through the world of psychiatry. In 1922, Hans Prinzhorn published *Artistry of the Mentally Ill*, based on the art of mentally ill people in asylums. This inspired two psychiatrists, Erich Guttmann and Francis Reitman, who emigrated to England from the Nazi persecution in the 1930s, to join with Walter Maclay to make a further collection of paintings for research. Edward Adamson was appointed as artist at the Netherne Hospital, with a brief to facilitate mentally ill patients in drawing and painting without any intervention. In this way he pioneered the 'open studio' approach (Adamson 1984).

A third strand was developed by Adrian Hill, who was the first person to use the term 'art therapy' in his book *Art Versus Illness* (1945). He had used his art to pass the time while convalescing from TB in 1938, and was then asked by doctors to help others, especially soldiers returning from the Second World War. It became apparent that 'doing art' achieved more than filling the hours – people actually recovered from their mental distress.

Many other pioneers were involved in the early days of art therapy, often working as artists, teachers or occupational therapists. They came together to form the British Association of Art Therapists (BAAT) in 1963. In the early days of BAAT there were strong links with teaching, but as art therapists found themselves increasingly working in hospitals BAAT looked more towards the NHS, achieving recognition in 1982. State registration was achieved in 1997 and from 1 April 2002 art therapists are registered by the Health Professions Council (HPC). (For addresses of BAAT and HPC see Resources section at end of book.) The two books concerning the history of art therapy in Britain are *Healing Arts* by Susan Hogan (2001), covering 1790 to 1966, and *Becoming a Profession* by Diane Waller (1991), covering 1940 to 1982.

Now art therapists work in a wide variety of settings. There is still a preponderance of art therapists working in mental health, but with the gradual closure of large hospitals they now work mostly in small hospitals or community mental health teams. Within the mental health system, art therapists work with those suffering from all kinds of disorders and at all stages of life. Art therapists now also work in forensic settings (prisons, regional secure units and youth offending teams) and in education (special needs schools, ordinary schools). There has been a growth of work in palliative care (cancer care, hospices, AIDS facilities), in addictions work (both alcohol and drugs) and in work with people with learning disabilities and those with autistic spectrum disorders. New areas are being explored all the time: art therapy with refugees and with children in war-torn zones are recent applications, where the aim is to bring appropriate relief in these situations. Several centres for homeless people also offer art therapy for their members or residents.

The non-verbal and creative aspects of art therapy make it the 'treatment of choice' (along with other arts therapies) for many who would not benefit from verbal therapies. In settings that include people with a wide range of abilities (both intellectual and emotional), it can be more inclusive of this diversity.

Art therapists undertake postgraduate training, lasting two years full time or three years part time. For those who do not want to train as art therapists but would like to find out more about it experientially, there is now a good range of introductory and foundation courses based at local colleges and some spring and summer schools based at universities, especially those engaged in art therapy training.

Arts therapists work from a variety of theoretical viewpoints, such as psychoanalytic (e.g. Freudian, Jungian, Kleinian) or humanistic (e.g. Gestalt, brief therapy, solution-focused, personal construct psychology, cognitive). Many arts therapists work in an eclectic way, selecting from different approaches; or use more than one approach, depending on the client group and the work to be done. One of the strengths of art therapy is that it can be used in conjunction with most psychological models.

Art therapy: some benefits

The following are some of the advantages of art therapy that may be relevant in different circumstances:

- Almost everyone has used art as a child and can still do so if encouraged to forget about images having to be 'artistically correct'.
- It can be used as a means of non-verbal communication. This can be important for those who do not have a good mastery of verbal communication for whatever reason. For those who cannot stop talking, it can sometimes be a good way of cutting through 'tangled verbosity'.

- It can be used as a means of self-expression and self-exploration. A picture is often a more precise description of feelings than words and can be used to depict experiences which are 'hard to put into words'. Sometimes 'words are hard to find', as in dementia. The spatial character of pictures can describe many aspects of experience simultaneously.
- The process of doing art can sometimes help people become more aware of feelings previously hidden from them, or of which they were only partly aware. It can help people become clearer about confused feelings.
- Using art can sometimes help people release feelings, e.g. anger and aggression, and can provide a safe and acceptable way of dealing with unacceptable feelings.
- It can help such people to look at their current situations and at ways of making changes. The 'framed experience' (an experience within a boundary, like a picture in a frame) can provide a context to try out or fantasise about possible futures without the commitment of reality.
- It can be used to help adults play and 'let go'. Recapturing the ability to play can lead to creativity and health.
- The concreteness of the products makes it easier to develop discussion from them. The pictures are there to return to at a later date and it is possible to look back over pictures from a series of sessions and note developments.
- The existence of a picture as a separate entity means that therapist and client can relate to each other through looking at the picture together. This is sometimes a less threatening way of confronting issues or relating. This is also referred to as the 'triangular relationship of art therapy'.
- Discussion of the products can lead to explorations of important issues. 'Interpretation' of a reductive kind is not widely used as pictures are often ambiguous and the most important thing is for the creator to find his or her own meanings.
- Using art requires active participation, which can help to mobilise people who have become accustomed to doing very little. In a group setting, it is one way of equalising participation. Everyone can join in at the same time and at their own level.
- It can be enjoyable and this may lead to shared pleasure and to individuals developing a sense of their own creativity. Many people who start art therapy in a very tentative way go on to develop a real interest in art.
- For certain disorders, it can be used diagnostically.

Art therapy can be used in many different ways, depending on the setting, the client group, the purpose and orientation of the therapist. As it has grown and been found useful in such a wide variety of situations, it can be practised in many different ways.

Art therapy and diversity

Art therapy and personal art groups have something particularly positive to offer in this area, as mentioned above, in that their non-verbal nature can include a wider diversity of clients than purely verbal therapies. The visual possibilities inherent in the use of art provide an exciting way to explore culture and difference. In areas such as this, questions are often more useful than hard-and-fast answers in that they open up areas for reflection and discussion. Campbell *et al.* (1999) explore this dimension in *Art Therapy, Race and Culture* and include the following questions in the Introduction:

1. How does the race and culture of both therapist and client impact on the process, product and relationships in art therapy?
2. How can we harness the therapeutic possibilities generated by images, colour and language, which reflect people's racial and cultural histories?
3. What are the content and meanings of the dynamics that arise in inter-cultural art therapy?

(Campbell *et al.* 1999: 15)

These questions can inform our explorations of race and culture and also of other areas of difference such as learning disabilities, gender, religion, and so on.

Art therapy and art activities

Although art therapists have forged the way, there are now many professionals who are interested in using art in a personal way with their groups. Many art courses and community arts programmes include a more personal approach to involvement in art. In art the emphasis is generally on the final product as an end in itself, whereas in art therapy the person and the process of creating the work are more important. However, with the more personal approaches in art there can be large overlaps. Many organisations now run arts activities which look quite similar to art therapy; for instance, mask workshops based on self-identity, group collages on the feelings of homeless people.

Art therapy and art activities are both valid processes in their own right, with different emphases. An art activity usually has as its aim the production of a picture, collage or sculpture, often involving a group. The aim is the completion of the work (and often its exhibition), but along the way participants often gain great benefit. Art therapy has as its aim the exploration of a personal problem or situation using art materials, but along the way art works of great merit may be produced. If we think of art therapy and art activities as ends of a continuum, then there will be many intermediate situations as well.

The exercises, themes and suggestions in this book can be used, with discretion, in a wide variety of situations, both in art therapy settings and in other settings where personal art activities are appropriate. It is up to the therapist or facilitator to make the judgements of appropriateness.

Why use groupwork?

For some facilitators and therapists there is a choice between individual work and groupwork, so it is worth looking at the general reasons for using groupwork. Others, such as teachers and community workers almost always work with groups and for them the important thing is to maximise the advantages groupwork can have. The reasons for using groupwork can be summarised as follows:

1 Much of social learning is done in groups; therefore groupwork provides a relevant context in which to practise.
2 People with similar needs can provide mutual support for each other and help with mutual problem solving.
3 Group members can learn from the feedback from other members.
4 Group members can try new roles, from seeing how others react (role modelling), and can be supported and reinforced in this.
5 Groupwork often brings up early family dynamics, which can then be examined and worked on.
6 Groups can be catalysts for developing latent resources and abilities.
7 Groups are more suitable for certain individuals, e.g. those who find the intimacy of individual work too intense.
8 Groups can be more democratic, sharing power and responsibility.
9 Some therapists/group workers find groupwork more satisfying than individual work.
10 Groups can be an economical way of using expertise to help several people at the same time.

However, there are also some disadvantages:

1 Confidentiality is more difficult because more people are involved.
2 Groups need resources and can be difficult to organise.
3 Less individual attention is available to members of a group.
4 A group may be 'labelled' or acquire a stigma.
5 People can more easily 'hide' or avoid issues.
6 Some participants may be intimidated by others' skills (Brown 1992: 13–16; Lumley-Smith 2002).

Why use art?

As well as the general points about the value of art therapy and personal art, there are some particular aspects that apply to groupwork:

1   It provides an activity that all can engage in. This is helpful for groups where some members find it difficult to talk, for whatever reason.
2   It provides a way of equalising participation in a group; everyone can join in at the same time at their own level.
3   It is possible to include a wider range of people than in a verbal group.
4   Participants see other members' pictures (and in some groups comment on them), and this provides a different dimension from a purely verbal group.
5   There is the possibility of using group interactive art exercises.
6   Using art generates a lot of material and this often accelerates group processes and dynamics.

Survey of art therapists

Many of the points mentioned above are relevant to groups working with art and were borne out in a survey I undertook in 1978 for my MA dissertation (Liebmann 1979). For this survey, I interviewed art therapists working in a wide variety of treatment and educational settings: general psychiatric and day hospitals, probation and social services day centres, schools, adolescent units, art therapy colleges, adult education institutes. They were working with an even wider cross-section of the community: long-stay and elderly patients, people with acute psychiatric crises, mental health patients, people with learning disabilities, ex-offenders, social work clients, people with alcohol problems, families, children, art therapists and social workers in training. I asked all the therapists what purposes their groups had and the answers seemed to fall into two clusters: personal and social. These are summarised in Tables 1.1 and 1.2.

As the tables show, art therapists saw their groups as aiming to enhance and sometimes change the personal and social functioning of the group members, rather than as a specific treatment for a particular disease.

There has been considerable research into therapeutic factors in groups in general. In her book *Group Interactive Art Therapy*, written after my research, Diane Waller (1993) summarises the generally agreed therapeutic factors of psychotherapy groups (Table 1.3).

Interestingly, the therapeutic factors from my survey and Diane Waller's summary are very similar to the therapeutic factors highlighted by Irvin Yalom in his well-known book *The Theory and Practice of Group Psychotherapy* (1995: 1).

Table 1.1   General personal purposes of groups

1.   Creativity and spontaneity
2.   Confidence building, self-validation, realisation of own potential
3.   Increase personal autonomy and motivation, develop as individual
4.   Freedom to make decisions, experiment, test out ideas
5.   Express feelings, emotions, conflicts
6.   Work with fantasy and unconscious
7.   Insight, self-awareness, reflection
8.   Ordering of experience visually and verbally
9.   Relaxation

Sources: Liebmann (1979: 27; 1981: 27; 1984: 159).

Table 1.2   General social purposes of groups

1.   Awareness, recognition, and appreciation of others
2.   Co-operation, involvement in group activity
3.   Communication
4.   Sharing of problems, experiences and insights
5.   Discovery of universality of experience/uniqueness of individual
6.   Relate to others in a group, understanding of effect of self on others, and relationships
7.   Social support and trust
8.   Cohesion of group
9.   Examine group issues

Sources: Liebmann (1979: 27; 1981: 27; 1984: 159).

Table 1.3   Therapeutic factors of psychotherapy groups

1.   Giving and sharing of information
2.   Instillation of hope
3.   Patients help each other
4.   Patients discover that others have the same problems, anxieties and fears
5.   The small group acts as a reconstruction of the family
6.   Catharsis – expression can bring great relief
7.   People can learn how they interact with others and have some feedback about this
8.   Group cohesiveness – it can be a safe place to share
9.   Interpersonal learning – old patterns can be examined and reworked

Source: Waller (1993: 35–6).

This enhancement of personal and social functioning is obviously applicable in a wide variety of settings, whether social, educational or therapeutic, and many include almost anyone who can function independently. Nor do these aims have to be confined to those labelled as in need of special help; they are human qualities we are all striving for, at one time or another. In fact, many of the art therapists I interviewed ran workshops for people in the wider community who wanted to explore themselves and their feelings and enhance their personal skills in dealing with these.

The importance of the list of therapeutic factors in Table 1.3 is that therapists and facilitators can think about which ones they consider particularly important for their client groups, and plan their groups to take account of them. For instance, if group cohesiveness is seen as important a therapist will want to take steps to ensure that group members understand the importance of attending all (or most of) the sessions.

Different styles of art therapy groupwork

Art therapy groups and personal art groups can provide a combination of individual and group experiences that draw on the traditions of both groupwork and art therapy. When I wrote the first edition of this book, it was the first book solely about art therapy groups and only the second published art therapy book in the UK. The situation is very different now. Several books and many chapters have been written about art therapy work with groups, describing and developing different ways of working.

Thinking about groupwork in general, there is an infinite variety of styles and modes, and many systems for trying to classify them: by client group; by aims; by theoretical basis; by practice method; by practical usefulness (Brown 1992: 19). Another classification could be by length of time. Even within group psychotherapy, Whitaker (2001: 60–1) quotes two classifications of psychotherapy groups, one with 10 types and one with 13 types. So it is not easy to set out a coherent typology.

I have tried to identify the main approaches that have emerged in the practice of art therapy groups, from my own knowledge and from the expanding literature. I have listed them in historical order of emergence in the literature (which may not be the same as their actual historical emergence). As far as I know, they are all in use at the time of writing. For each approach I have given one or two references; a more comprehensive listing of books including art therapy with groups is given in the Resources section at the end of the book. It is not always easy to see each approach as completely distinct as they sometimes overlap or 'borrow' from each other.

Open studio approach

Group members meet in the same room to draw and paint, each person getting on with their own work at their own pace. Any sharing of the work is done individually with the therapist. The atmosphere is informal and relaxed. The group does not come together for any discussion. This was historically the first kind of art therapy group and is still used for low-key, long-term art therapy groups where painting together with others is important but a formal or interactive group would be too stressful (Adamson 1984; Deco 1998). One organisation currently specialising in this approach is Studio Upstairs: 'a unique therapeutic community for those whose talents and interests can be expressed through the arts, but who may be too vulnerable to participate in the traditional artistic institutions . . .

Members work side by side, and a flexible approach is taken to meet individual needs' (Studio Upstairs 2002; see Resources section for address).

Theme-based groups

These groups meet for a common purpose to look at particular problems or aspects of human experience; e.g. bereavement, anger, life transitions. This way of working is particularly suited to short-life groups that come together for this specific purpose. It is also useful for single-session groups that are part of a longer programme; e.g. an alcohol education group which involves mostly verbal work but includes one art session; Bristol Cancer Help Centre, where the art therapy session is part of a two-day single visit to the centre. It can also help to introduce art therapy to people who are unfamiliar with it; i.e. for the first few sessions of a group before members develop their own themes. There is usually a formal structure to the group, with an introduction, the choice of a theme (by the therapist or group members), and a time for group members to draw or paint, followed by a time of sharing (Barber 2002; Campbell 1993; Liebmann 2004; Ross 1997). Sometimes themes develop out of members' discussion at the beginning of a session (Greenwood and Layton 1987; Liebmann 2002, 2004).

Group analytic art groups

This way of working has been developed particularly by Gerry McNeilly and is outlined in several articles (1984, 1987, 1989, 2000). In these groups there is no set direction or topic and the aim is for the group to explore and treat itself. The group analytic approach is based on the work of Foulkes: 'Group analysis is analysis of the group, by the group, including the conductor' (Foulkes 1983). Thus the emphasis is on 'here and now' under-standings of the whole group, including the conductor (McNeilly 1989: 157). Even though no topic is set, often there is a resonance of themes in the artwork of group members, usually related to internal or external events, e.g. a therapist leaving (McNeilly 1984; Roberts 1985).

Group interactive art therapy

These groups have been described by Diane Waller (1993); she draws on group analytic insights and some theme-based work to provide art therapy groups where the focus is both on individual artwork and the group dynamics between group members. Thus the group can be an important arena for learning about personal relationships (Waller 1993).

Art psychotherapy groups

The book of this title (Skaife and Huet 1998) looks particularly at the way art-making can enable a group psychodynamic therapeutic process to take place which would be difficult with a purely verbal psychotherapy group. The authors also consider the dilemmas arising between the verbal interaction and the art-making (Skaife and Huet 1998: 14). The book extends the theoretical exploration and applications to different client groups (Skaife and Huet 1998).

Art-based groups exploring social and life issues

To some extent this might be included under theme-based groups, but there has been a recent burgeoning of arts-based work with many groups, especially those for whom talking and writing have not been productive. Examples of these are: work with conflict issues (Liebmann 1996); murals with young people (Linfield and van Loock 2002); spiritual issues (Cook and Heales 2001); work with asylum seekers (Deyes 2002), and many others. Some of these are facilitated by artists or artists in residence schemes, while for others the organisers search out art therapists because of their skills in working with vulnerable people.

There has been considerable debate concerning the merits of all these approaches to art therapy groups, and at times this became quite heated. But there is now more acceptance that this is a subject on which different views exist and may be shared. In fact, this 'typology' is not a watertight classification. Some authors describe art therapy groups that include features from several of the above types of group. Many art therapists also work in different ways with different groups. It is up to each group facilitator or therapist to decide which approach suits their group and situation best, and what training and preparation they need before undertaking such work.

Why use themes?

This book is concerned with the second type of art therapy groupwork, in which groups meet to share a common task or explore a common theme. Some of the reasons for using themes and exercises are given below. It is worth reflecting on them to see if they apply to your group:

1   Many people have great difficulty in starting. A theme can give a focus to begin somewhere.
2   Some initial themes can help groups understand what art therapy is all about. This is especially true if people in the group are not familiar with the approach and see the art group only in terms of former school art lessons or external aesthetic standards.

3   Some groups include people who are very insecure and need some structure if they are to operate at all.
4   There is often pressure of time. For community groups and training courses, the art group may be only one session, a day, or a weekend. Even in hospitals and day centres, many people only stay a short time, in order to return to normal life as quickly as possible. A group can get to the point more quickly if it focuses on a suitable theme.
5   Sharing a theme can help to weld a group together.
6   Themes and exercises can be interpreted on many levels and used flexibly to meet different needs. The group can be involved in the choice of theme if this is appropriate.
7   Certain themes can be useful in helping members of the group to relate to each other.
8   Sometimes themes can help people to get out of 'ruts' by facilitating work and discussion which would otherwise not happen (Liebmann 1979, 1985, 1986; Thornton 1985).

Using themes to the best advantage presupposes all the experience and preparation mentioned in the Introduction. If used inappropriately, some themes can evoke feelings which are too much for that group to handle at that time. At the other end of the spectrum, some can lead to a superficial experience which leaves people dissatisfied. Between these two poles there is a wide variety of group experiences using art-based themes which can be interesting and revealing and also enjoyable.

Flexible use of themes

Many groups will use both sessions of theme-based work and sessions in which everyone 'does their own thing'. Figure 1.1 shows the continuum of possibilities (Liebmann 1979: 28).

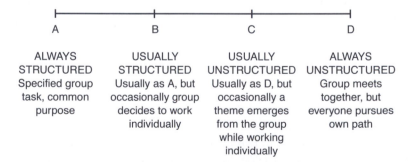

Figure 1.1   Continuum of possibilities for work in art therapy groups
Source: Liebmann (1986)

Working in a 'theme-based' way can mean many things. It can mean using just a simple boundary rule such as 'Paint what you like, but use only three colours' or it can mean a more prescribed activity such as 'Choose one crayon and have a non-verbal conversation with another person on the same piece of paper'. Again, there is a continuum from instructions which are so loose that they do not constitute a theme at all to activities which could be described as very specific themes (Liebmann 1979). This can be illustrated by looking at some different possible introductions:

1   We are going to 'do our own thing'.
2   Use a large sheet of paper and your three favourite colours to draw a picture of anything you like.
3   Start with a doodle and see if it turns into anything.
4   Paint a childhood incident.
5   Paint a childhood incident which was a turning point.
6   Paint your first experience of separation.
7   Paint your first day at school.

The first one is obviously not a theme, although even to say 'Do your own thing' is a certain kind of structure. The second and third provide a minimal theme as a start but do not specify anything further. The last four are recognisably 'themes' and progressively more specific. It is sometimes worth being fairly specific if the aim is to share common experiences, but not so specific that there is no room for individual choice and interpretation of the theme, at whatever level is appropriate. So, for a group of adults, the last one on the list might be too specific as it does not leave room for anyone who cannot or does not want to remember their first day at school.

Useful themes are usually flexible enough to allow for many levels of response. Starting with a particular theme, we can develop it by adding to it or changing it, and see how this changes the activity and its meaning. It is easier to see how this might work if we look at a practical example. For instance, the theme 'Draw an advertisement for yourself' can be interpreted on several different levels. It could be an opportunity to display or acknowledge one's best points (which modesty and our self-deprecating culture often do not allow); or to discover some new assets in the process of doing the picture; or to learn about others; or to select qualities which appeal to certain kinds of other people (as advertisements are aimed at particular targets); or to consider whether we are different with different kinds of people.

Then we could also develop it. When each person has drawn their own self-advertisement, others in the group add qualities that have been missed; or the group members can select from others' 'wares' or 'trade' them. There are many possibilities. All these changes will produce an effect that will make it a different activity. Most of the changes suggested here make the activity more interactive, which is only possible if all or most join in. Many personal themes can be developed into group interaction in this way. See Part II, Section I (group interactive exercises) and compare, for instance, how theme 138 (Metaphorical Portraits) can be changed into a group interactive exercise (286).

One of the most valuable qualities of art therapy and personal art is the provision of a parallel frame of reference to real life, in which different ways of being can be tried out without any real-life consequences. Small risks can be attempted before large ones. Perhaps someone doing the Advertisement exercise might be helped by group members to acknowledge some good qualities. The next step, in the day-to-day world, might be to let others know about these good qualities, instead of hiding them.

The structure of some themes can provide a useful non-literal frame of reference. An example of this might be the use made of the Metaphorical Portraits game at a day workshop (see Chapter 6, Example 21), where one woman drew another as a brick wall with a green tree peeping out behind (see Figure 6.14). Here the structure of the interactive theme provided a framework which made it possible for them to refer, in a non-literal way, to their difficult relationship in a way they had not been able to before. The presence of the tree signified hope and change and the two women were able to discuss this, leading to a fresh start in communicating with each other.

Conclusion

This chapter has given an overview of art therapy and developments in art therapy groups and provided some frameworks to the reasons for using themes in art therapy groups. It has looked at the contribution that flexible theme-based work can make. This forms a useful background in thinking about groups before embarking on the practical steps of running a group, which is the topic of the next chapter.

References

Adamson, E. (1984) *Art as Healing*, London: Coventure.

Barber, V. (2002) *Explore Yourself Through Art: Creative Projects to Promote Personal Insight, Growth and Problem-solving*, London: Carroll & Brown.

Brown, A. (1992) *Groupwork*, 3rd edn, Aldershot: Ashgate.

Campbell, J. (1993) *Creative Art in Groupwork*, Bicester: Speechmark.

Campbell, J., Liebmann, M., Brooks, F., Jones, J. and Ward, C. (eds) (1999) *Art Therapy, Race and Culture*, London: Jessica Kingsley Publishers.

Case, C. and Dalley, T. (1992) *The Handbook of Art Therapy*, London: Tavistock/ Routledge.

Cook, C. and Heales, B.C. (2001) *Seeding the Spirit: The Appleseed Workbook*, Birmingham: Woodbrooke Quaker Study Centre.

Deco, S. (1998) 'Return to the open studio group: art therapy groups in acute psychiatry', in S. Skaife and V. Huet (eds) *Art Psychotherapy Groups*, London: Routledge.

Deyes, T. (2002) 'Asylum seekers: unravelling the knot', *Mailout*, June/July: 6–8.

Foulkes, S.H. (1983) *Introduction to Group Analytic Psychotherapy*, Croydon: Medway Press.

Greenwood, H. and Layton, G. (1987) 'An out patient art therapy group', *Inscape*, Summer: 12–19.

Hill, A. (1945) *Art Versus Illness*, London: George, Allen & Unwin.

Hogan, S. (2001) *Healing Arts: The History of Art Therapy*, London: Jessica Kingsley Publishers.

Liebmann, M. F. (1979) 'A study of structured art therapy groups', unpublished MA thesis, Birmingham Polytechnic.

Liebmann, M. F. (1981) 'The many purposes of art therapy', *Inscape*, 5, 1: 26–8.

Liebmann, M. F. (1984) 'Art games and group structures', in T. Dalley (ed.) *Art as Therapy*, London: Tavistock.

Liebmann, M. F. *et al.* (1985) Letter to *Inscape*, late issue 1: 25.

Liebmann, M. F. (1986) *Art Therapy for Groups*, 1st edn, London: Croom Helm.

Liebmann, M. F. (1996) *Arts Approaches to Conflict*, London: Jessica Kingsley Publishers.

Liebmann, M. F. (2002) 'Developing games, activities, and themes for art therapy groups', in C. A. Malchiodi (ed.) *Handbook of Art Therapy*, London: Guilford Press.

Liebmann, M. F. (2004) *Art Therapy for Groups*, 2nd edn, Hove: Brunner-Routledge.

Linfield, N. and van Loock, D. (2002) 'Youth art: working on a mural with young people', unpublished report.

Lumley-Smith, E. (2002) Personal communication.

McNeilly, G. (1984) 'Directive and non-directive approaches in art therapy', *Inscape*, December: 7–12.

McNeilly, G. (1987) 'Further contributions to group analytic art therapy', *Inscape*, Summer: 8–11.

McNeilly, G. (1989) 'Group analytic art groups', in A. Gilroy and T. Dalley (eds) *Pictures at an Exhibition*, London: Tavistock/Routledge.

McNeilly, G. (2000) 'Failure in group analytic art therapy', in A. Gilroy and G. McNeilly (eds) *The Changing Shape of Art Therapy*, London: Jessica Kingsley Publishers.

Payne, H. (1993) *Handbook of Inquiry in the Arts Therapies: One River, Many Currents*, London: Jessica Kingsley Publishers.

Prinzhorn, H. (1922) *Bildernei der Geisteskrank*, Berlin: Springer Verlag; trans. E. von Brockendorff (1972) *Artistry of the Mentally Ill*, Berlin: Springer Verlag.

Roberts, J. P. (1985) 'Resonance in art groups', *Inscape*, late issue 1: 17–20.

Ross, C. (1997) *Something to Draw On: Activities and Interventions using an Art Therapy Approach*, London: Jessica Kingsley Publishers.

Skaife, S. and Huet, V. (eds) (1998) *Art Psychotherapy Groups*, London: Routledge.

Studio Upstairs (2002) *Annual Report 2001*, London: Studio Upstairs.

Thornton, R. (1985) 'A critique', *Inscape*, late issue 1: 23–5.

Waller, D. (1991) *Becoming a Profession: The History of Art Therapy in Britain 1940–82*, London: Tavistock/Routledge.

Waller, D. (1993) *Group Interactive Art Therapy: Its Use in Training and Treatment*, London: Routledge.

Whitaker, D. S. (2001) *Using Groups to Help People*, 2nd edn, London: Brunner-Routledge.

Yalom, I. D. (1995) *The Theory and Practice of Group Psychotherapy*, 4th edn, New York: Basic Books.

Chapter 2

Running a group

Before starting on some of the practicalities of running a group, it is worth remembering that the whole purpose of the group is to provide a warm, trusting environment in which people can feel at ease in revealing personal matters. Caring and respect for other people, and for their feelings and points of view are a priority. The suggestions given in this chapter are designed to help to achieve this kind of caring, client-centred group which people enjoy being in. There are several points to think about in relation to running a group and a checklist of them is useful:

1 Setting up the group
2 Equal opportunities
3 Outside factors affecting the group
4 Aims and goals
5 Group boundaries and ground rules
6 Size of group
7 Open and closed groups
8 Therapist and facilitator roles
9 Transference and projections
10 Usual pattern for session
11 Alternative patterns of sessions
12 Introductions and 'warming up'
13 Choosing a theme
14 Engaging in the artwork
15 Discussion
16 Interpretation
17 Ending the session
18 Group process over time
19 Recording and evaluation

The rest of the chapter will look briefly at each of these aspects in turn. For further information on groupwork, please see Resources section.

Setting up the group

This is often the hardest part and requires a good deal of time and energy to achieve. The following points need to be worked out and settled.

Therapist(s) or facilitator(s)

- Are there suitable and experienced therapists/facilitators for this group or workshop?
- Does there need to be a co-therapist or facilitator?
- What are the arrangements for supervision?
- Is payment involved?
- What is the insurance provision?

Room

- Is there a suitable room and is it large enough?
- How will you gain access when you run your group?
- Is the room wheelchair accessible?
- Where are the toilets in relation to the room?
- Where is the designated smoking area, and is it inside or outside the building?
- Is the room light enough in daylight or artificial light?
- Is there access to a sink and water?
- Are there tables and chairs?
- Is there enough floor space for what you want to do?
- Is there room for paintings to dry?
- Where will you hold discussions of work done?
- Will the room dictate using dry media only?
- Will the room be quiet enough?
- Do you need facilities to make drinks or serve food?
- Where is the first aid box and is it complete?
- Where are the fire exits and where is the gathering point in case of fire?
- How can you access help in case of emergencies?
- Is there a telephone or do you need to bring a mobile phone?
- Are there any other health and safety issues?

Time

- Is there a suitable slot on the institutional timetable?
- What activities will come before and after which might influence the art session?
- If it is a single session, such as an evening or day workshop, which day and what time are best?

Materials

Which of the materials listed below do you want to include? (See also section M, Media Notes, at end of book.)

- paints – powder paints, blocks or redimix liquid paints (the latter are easier to use and need no preparation); for some groups, fluorescent and metallic colours have an appeal
- utensils for handling paint, e.g. spoons for powder paint, wire for freeing blocked liquid paint containers (large paper clips are useful for this)
- palettes for holding paints and mixing them (yoghurt trays from supermarkets can be useful as disposable palettes); plastic trays for larger amounts
- water containers
- brushes – large, medium and small
- sponges and rollers – for large paintings and a different experience from brushes
- dry media – soft (e.g. 2B) pencils, coloured pencils, wax crayons, felt-tip pens, oil pastels, conté crayons, charcoal, water-soluble crayons
- paper – sugar paper, lining paper, cartridge paper, newsprint rolls; different colours and sizes
- card – thin or thick – for three-dimensional work
- clay and boards (and some means of keeping clay damp and cool; also some means of cutting individual lumps off such as cheese-wire or a strong knife); stoneware and earthenware clay need a kiln for firing; newclay is self-hardening (nylon-reinforced) and can be painted
- plasticine and other modelling materials (for playdough, see no. 75 for recipes)
- collage materials – magazines, textured materials, fabrics, coloured tissue paper, string, natural objects, glitter, sequins, etc.
- junk materials for 3-D work, e.g. boxes, wire, pipecleaners, found objects
- scissors (sharp but round tipped), craft knives, ordinary strong knives (select with regard for client group and safety issues)
- adhesives – glue for collage (PVA is useful) and three-dimensional work (stronger glue), sellotape, masking tape
- rags and paper tissues or kitchen roll for wiping up
- newspaper or polythene sheet to cover up tables or carpet or for paintings to dry on
- old shirts or cheap plastic aprons to protect clothes (or ask people to wear old clothes).

Many of these items will need buying or ordering well in advance, especially if you work in an institution that orders all its equipment from certain suppliers. Many towns and cities now have a 'scrapstore', resources centre or similar project that recycles industrial offcuts to schools, hospitals and other helping organisations. They often have good supplies of paper, card and plastic containers and sometimes also buy in a range of cheap art materials. Art materials can be ordered at reasonable prices (cheaper than retailers) from a number of catalogues. Details of scrapstores and catalogues can be found in the Resources section at the end of the book.

Members of group

This is probably the most tricky of all. You may need a referral system, which you will need to explain to other staff. How can they easily know who is going to benefit from the art group you are going to run? You may need to talk to other staff about the sort of 'ready-made' groups (e.g. a ward, a class, an elderly persons' home) which would gain from regular art therapy or personal art sessions. One good way of introducing this activity is to have a workshop for other staff first so that they have a first-hand knowledge of what is involved and also have a chance to ask questions about any misgivings they may have. If you are working in an institution, it is important to get as much support as possible for what you are doing before you start.

If you are intending to run a limited length group around a particular theme you will need to write a page or leaflet about it, with details of how staff can refer clients or clients can refer themselves. This information needs to contain practical details (time, place, duration, facilitators) and something about the purpose of the group, its ethos, expectations (e.g. drop-in or attend every session) and how it will operate.

For formal therapy groups an interview or preparatory session is a good idea. This is a chance for therapists to check that clients are suitable and prepared for the realities of the group and for clients to check that the group is for them. It can also start the trust-building process between clients and therapist(s), so that the first session is not quite so daunting for clients.

If you are running a workshop for members of the community (e.g. a day workshop for people working in the caring professions), you will need to think about posters and how to word them to attract those you want (and perhaps deflect those you do not feel you can cope with). You will need to leave plenty of time for publicity and also to think about costs and payment.

Equal opportunities

Most organisations have an equal opportunities policy that sets out policy toward minority groups, discrimination and access to services. In practice this means keeping in mind the following considerations:

1   There should be no discrimination on grounds of race, ethnic back-
     ground, culture, religion, gender, sexual orientation, class, disability or
     age. The exception to this is 'positive discrimination' in provision for
     minority groups, such as 'elderly Asian clients' group' or 'young gay
     people's group'. Sometimes group applicants may find themselves 'in a
     minority of one', e.g. the only black person or the only woman. In such
     cases it may be advisable to check with that person whether she or he is
     happy to join the group under those conditions, or whether it would be
     too stressful and a wait for the next group would be preferable. What
     support might they need to participate in the group (e.g. facilitators
     being alert to the issues, perhaps including 'no sexist or racist language'
     in the ground rules, etc.)? A preliminary interview can be an oppor-
     tunity to ask applicants about these things.

2   The group venue should be easily accessible in terms of transport
     (public transport, car parking, safe place for bikes), social and physical
     needs (safety, area of town, time of day) and in terms of access to the
     building (steps, stairs, toilets). In practice this is difficult for many
     organisations, but from October 2004 the Disability Discrimination
     Act 1995 places a duty on all public service providers to make 'reas-
     onable adjustments' to physical features of their premises to overcome
     physical barriers to access (DRC 2002: 4–6). An 'access audit' can help
     here (DRC 2002: 39–40, 50). DIAL (Disability Information Advice
     Line) UK can provide contact details of local centres with information
     about accessible venues and other disability information (see Resources
     section).

3   There may be a need for interpreters for some or all members of a
     group. This may be for mother-tongue languages for non-English
     speakers or for sign language for deaf people. Even if the group
     members in question speak some English, it may be important to have
     an interpreter as subtle emotions may only be expressible in people's
     own languages. It will usually be necessary to book interpreters well
     ahead and it is important to use properly accredited interpreters and
     agencies rather than informal arrangements. It is important to discuss
     what you need the interpreter to do before the group starts. They
     should only translate, not pass opinions or join in the group and not
     have 'side conversations' inaccessible to the rest of the group. A point
     to watch for is confidentiality, especially if the minority is a small one
     where everyone knows each other. It is also worth asking whether a
     particular interpreter is acceptable, in case she/he is from a group which
     is in conflict with your client's group. Finally – check that the inter-
     preter speaks the right language!

4   It is important to be aware of language, both in written material about
     the group and within the group in spoken language. This can be
     included in ground rules (see Group Boundaries and Ground Rules

section of this chapter). Facilitators need to be ready to challenge members' use of racist or sexist language (for example) in a constructive way, such as by reminding group members of the ground rules, or asking whether a stereotype is actually true. Vicky Barber and Jean Campbell (1999) discuss the layers of meaning involved in using the word 'black' in an art therapy group, as it can indicate paint, people or politics – with neutral, positive or negative associations. In a group that I ran a man came out with some sexist language about the roles of women and men concerning housework: 'I don't keep a dog and bark myself.' Instead of telling him off, I suggested, 'Let's check this out with the other men in the group – what are your views?' It turned out they undertook a variety of household tasks and it was clear to him that his views were not shared. Facilitators also need to be open to challenges from group members if they find any particular use of language upsetting or offensive.

5   It is good to try to avoid making assumptions and to question them if others make them, such as 'All men are . . .' or that people with a certain religion always act in a certain way. Often in a group this questioning of assumptions can lead to interesting discussion and opportunities for learning for all.

6   There may be some quite small adjustments that will make a difference to whether people with mild disabilities can take part with comfort; e.g. making sure that someone with partial hearing or sight is sitting in the best position in the group, providing thick pens for people with arthritis, checking whether people have knee problems before suggesting an exercise on the floor.

Rather than being seen as 'a burden of political correctness', paying attention to these factors should be seen as part of a creative journey to discover each other in our widest humanity (Campbell 1993: 23). My own experience in this area took off when I was no longer afraid to ask questions and was able to learn from the answers I received.

Outside factors affecting the group

These are the factors over which you may have no control, but which may affect your group. Many of them have been mentioned in the previous sections.

Institutional factors

Your group may be bound by institutional timetables such as mealtimes, times of transport, shift changes, break times, etc. It will also be affected by the amount of support there is for you and your kind of work; e.g. if there is little support you may be subject to interruptions or find group members suddenly withdrawn. If there is good support there will be respect for you and what your group needs, perhaps other staff helping and interest shown in the results. Sometimes there can be problems if the aims of the group are different from the aims of the institution, or if group members receive different messages from different therapists or staff members.

Physical factors

An art therapy group can be affected very much by the space at its disposal. Groups which have to take place in small, dark, claustrophobic rooms are restricted in what they can achieve – as are groups in rooms which are through routes to other rooms and subject to constant interruptions. Noise from adjacent rooms, lack of suitable tables and presence of unsuitable carpets can further inhibit groups. By contrast, a quiet, light room with a messy painting area and a comfortable discussion space can do much to enhance a group's experience.

Clientele

This will of course be the most important factor determining what you can and cannot expect to do with your group. Obviously, different groups will have different needs and be able to cope with different activities. You may be working with long-term rehabilitation ward patients in a hospital, ex-offenders in a day centre, children and young people in a 'special needs' group, a social services staff team, acute admissions patients in a psychiatric hospital, cancer patients in the community, elderly people attending a day centre or a group of adults with learning disabilities, to name but a few client groups. They may bring a wide variety of problems with them that need to be taken into account. Elderly and disabled people may need wheelchairs or have difficulty with vision and hearing; steps can sometimes be taken to help with these (e.g. chunky grips for pencils and crayons). Physically ill people may be very tired and in considerable pain, and therefore have limited concentration. Children, people with learning disabilities and some elderly patients with dementia may also have very short concentration spans. In any of these groups there may be a lot in common between members or a great mixture of sometimes incompatible people. There will be different levels of insight and awareness. Sometimes there may be inappropriate people present who can be disruptive.

Feelings

People arrive at a group session bringing with them feelings from all sorts of other situations, whether from the outside world or from elsewhere within an institution. They may be feeling flat, high, anxious, preoccupied or simply very tired. It is a good idea to check how people are feeling at the beginning of a session. This may influence your choice of activity or help you realise your opportunities or likely limitations to achievement that session. If an art therapy session does not go very well, it may not be because of what has happened in the group but because of something else that happened outside it. In some institutions the art therapy session is part of a planned programme (e.g. in many day centres), and you need to be aware of what has gone before.

Aims and goals

It is important to be clear about (at least some of) your aims and goals. It may help to look at the lists in Tables 1.1, 1.2 and 1.3 to see which aims and goals you have in mind for your group. You may have other aims which are important. Ask yourself why this group is coming together for a personal art or art therapy session. Here are a few examples of different aims:

- a group of psychiatric patients in hospital is exploring the factors precipitating their admission
- a group of workers in the helping professions may want to find out what art therapy is all about
- a women's group experiencing a 'sticky patch' is trying the use of art as a non-verbal means of communication
- an Asian women's group meets to explore how to cope better with anger and conflict
- a group of adults with learning disabilities is exploring their creativity
- a group of elderly people in a day centre is using the art group to reflect on their lives, both happy and unhappy events
- a single session for cancer patients aims to open some doors for them to explore further on their own
- a day workshop for a church group may seek to involve adults and children in activities which both can use equally well for meaningful communication
- a group of mediators attends a workshop to look at conflict issues through art
- a Jewish group meets to explore Holocaust issues through art.

(Note: some of the above groups are described in some detail in Chapter 6.)

Group boundaries and ground rules

Every group needs a few ground rules to know where it stands, and for members to know what is expected and (just as important) not expected.

Some of these will be worked out beforehand, such as whether there is a 'contract' to attend a certain number of sessions, and whether certain people need to be excluded (e.g. because previous experience has shown that they are disruptive and the group cannot operate properly with them in it). Others will need to be established when the group starts. Many of these will be implicitly assumed by those with group experience, but may need emphasising for those new to groupwork. Some need to be worked out with group members. Here are some to consider:

- *Normal social rules*: e.g. no interrupting, respect for others, arriving on time, etc.
- *Practical details if appropriate*: toilets, breaks, drinks, food, etc.
- *Importance of confidentiality*: the group needs to feel safe. In practice the precise meaning of confidentiality needs spelling out. A narrow definition is 'Everything said here stays here', whereas a wider definition might be 'Everyone is free to talk about general things and his or her own contribution, but not about others in any way that they could be recognised.'
- *Participation*: it is vital to let people know if they are expected to participate and to talk about their work, and also if this is not required.
- *Time limits*: these need to be spelled out, and whether people are expected to stay all the time, so that people can avoid being left with 'unfinished business' when the group ends.
- *Attendance*: in a closed group will people be expected to attend every session, and what will happen if they miss sessions?
- *Talking during the activity*: is this to be encouraged or discouraged? Many therapists and facilitators feel the experience of painting is more intense if there is no talking, but some use painting as a means of enabling talking to start.
- *Smoking*: many buildings are now no-smoking zones apart from special designated areas, so if there are smokers in the group arrangements need to be made for them to smoke during breaks if they need to. This is often outside, but smokers may need to go to the designated smoking area.
- *Mobile phones*: it is clearly best if these are firmly switched off during sessions. However occasionally there may be people (staff or members) who are expecting to be called in an emergency and the group will have to negotiate arrangements for the least disruption.
- *Facilitator participation*: decide whether you as facilitator are going to join in or not.
- *Group responsibility*: decide what this means. It may mean everyone being responsible for their own feelings; or everyone joining in the discussion; or everyone helping to choose the theme. It may also mean everyone helps with the clearing up!

Size of group

Most art therapy and personal art groups, in common with other small groups, have a membership of between 4 and 12, although larger groups are occasionally manageable. This size is important to ensure the following factors:

- Members can maintain visual and verbal contact with all other members.
- Group cohesiveness can be achieved.
- There is an opportunity for each person to have an adequate share of time in discussion.
- There are enough people to encourage interaction and a free flow of ideas, and to undertake group projects.

Smaller groups of six to eight are generally found to be more intimate and supportive, fulfilling the first three criteria, whereas larger groups may provide more interaction and creativity and 'somewhere to hide' if this is needed. Many groups also suffer from people dropping out, so if that is likely therapists and facilitators need to recruit two or three more participants than their ideal number. Groups that drop to very low numbers can be very hard work to maintain. (Benson 2001: 27–8; Brown 1992: 54–5; Whitaker 2001: 73–4).

Open and closed groups

One important decision to be made is whether the group is to be a closed or open group. A closed group usually runs for a fixed number of sessions with the same members. This means that members can get to know each other well and build up trust, to share at a deep level. An open group allows people to join and leave as they wish, and consequently remains at a fairly superficial level. Many groups in day hospitals and day centres are closed groups with a commitment to attend. However, groups for inpatients are more likely to be open groups, as patients are discharged as soon as possible to prevent disruption to their lives and institutionalisation.

Semi-open groups are a useful compromise. There is usually a commitment to attend but membership changes slowly as people leave and newcomers arrive. In this way the group ethos is maintained, while allowing for a natural or organised turnover. This kind of group is also usual in many day hospitals and day centres and also in many ongoing community groups.

For closed and semi-open groups in institutions there is often a referral and assessment procedure for clients, to check suitability and motivation and for clients to check if it is what they want to do. This can include a simple application form, an interview with the group facilitators, trying out some artwork or all of these. It may also involve taking part in a 'before the group' measurement for an evaluation.

Therapist and facilitator roles

There are many styles of facilitating a group and observation of other group facilitators and therapists is most helpful in deciding which style is suitable for you and your group. It is also worth consulting some books on groupwork. A few points are worth emphasising here.

Presence of a co-therapist or co-facilitator

This can be very valuable as it means there are two people to discuss how to run the group in the first place, and this can avoid many pitfalls. In the session itself a co-facilitator can provide a 'model' for group members, can support the lead facilitator and (if necessary) go and help a group member who leaves suddenly. This is very important in groups where there may be volatile or vulnerable members. After the session, two heads are better than one at evaluation. It is most important to work out the roles beforehand as there is nothing worse than two facilitators at cross-purposes. Having a co-facilitator in the anger management art therapy group (see Chapter 6) was vital as one or two members needed to leave the room if they felt in danger of 'blowing'.

Joining in

The decision on whether or not to join in with the group usually depends on the ethos of the group and the framework in which it takes place. Many facilitators and therapists join in the actual painting or other artwork because they feel that if they expect others to participate and to be open then they ought to set an example. In this way they are demonstrating that they are also members of the group, rather than aloof observers. Greenwood and Layton (1987, 1991) talk about 'side-by-side' therapy. However, there are also some very sound reasons for not joining in, such as concentrating on the organisation of materials for group members, being available to group members on an individual basis, or concentrating on observation where this is judged the most important task of the leader. This decision has to be an individual one, according to the setting, the needs of the group and the personal philosophy of the therapist or facilitator. If facilitators do participate, they need to ensure that they do not become so immersed in their own work that they fail to pay attention to the group, which is, after all, their primary task.

Group involvement

Some groups look very much to the facilitator, and this can be quite appropriate. The facilitator initiates the sessions and most of the comments are directed at her/him. In other groups, the facilitator consciously tries to involve the group as democratically as possible. Initially this may mean encouraging group members, in discussion time, to ask questions and make comments directly to other group members. As time goes on, members of the group may help to choose themes for the group and be more involved in the general running; e.g. in helping new members find their feet, etc. They may also relate more to other members.

Transference and projections

These are terms which are sometimes used by therapists to talk about groups with a psychotherapeutic orientation.

Transference

This describes the tendency of group members to 'transfer' feelings for significant figures in their lives on to the group facilitator or therapist. They may, for instance, 'project' their continued need for a parent on to the group facilitator or therapist. This may lead to over-dependence on him or her, or to conflict, according to previous experience. In institutions, this tendency is often enhanced by the fact that doctors and therapists are seen as having (and do in fact have) considerable power and authority.

For example, an art therapist working with a community group over several months (see Chapter 5), was approached by a group member with a request for individual therapy. She had become aware of his increasing dependence on her and suspected that he saw her in a parental role. This was confirmed for her when he asked her to be his individual therapist. She acknowledged his need, but felt it would be inappropriate for her to fulfil it and gave him the name of another therapist who was not involved with the group.

Countertransference

This usually refers to 'therapists' personal feelings and responses in a group which are rooted in her or his personal needs' (Whitaker 2001: 103). It may also mean responding to a transference from a group member as if he or she were that significant figure from the past, e.g. like the group member's parent. For example, a facilitator or therapist may find a certain group member particularly irritating. On reflection he or she may realise that this person has attributes that remind them of their own brother, sister or parent.

Identification

This is a process in which a person sees another as a similar or more ideal version of him or herself and changes by modelling himself or herself on these aspects (Case and Dalley 1992: 245). A group member may identify with a facilitator or with another group member. Group members identifying with each other can provide useful motivation and discussion, sometimes leading to change. For instance, two men attending an art therapy anger management group (see Chapter 6) found great comfort in each other's presence as their situations were similar. Both had 12-year-old sons and said their reasons for attending the group were to give them a better life than they had experienced. However, if the identification is too strong it can become restricting, as people need to work towards being more fully themselves rather than a clone of another person.

Projection

This is a process in which group members have feelings and make assumptions about other members not based on experience in the group. This can lead to them projecting their own attributes or feelings (while unaware of them) on to other participants. Sometimes this can lead to scapegoating of one member by all the others (Waller 1993: 24). The recipient of the projection or scapegoating can be a member or one of the therapists.

Other psychoanalytic terms

There is a useful glossary of psychoanalytic terms in *The Handbook of Art Therapy* (Case and Dalley 1992). If you are involved in a group in which therapists work with these concepts, you will probably already be involved in some further training in this connection. However, many groups neither use these terms nor make specific use of these concepts in their way of working. Nevertheless, it is worth being aware of what is happening, even if only to acknowledge it (see Chapter 4, Example 19) or to take appropriate action.

Usual pattern for session

The most usual format for a theme-based art therapy group is as follows (Liebmann 1979: 51–2):

1   Introduction and 'warming up': 10–30 minutes.
2   Artwork: 20–45 minutes.
3   Discussion of images: 30–45 minutes.
4   Ending: 5–10 minutes.

In many institutions the time available is one and a half to two hours and the timings given above fit into this. For community groups and professionals, longer times could be more appropriate with more time allowed for both the artwork and the discussion. The stages above will be explained in more detail below, together with some suggestions on how to choose an appropriate activity or theme. Of course, there are many other formats for sessions and some of these are now described.

Alternative patterns of sessions

Although very many personal art and art therapy groups use the format outlined in the last section, and much of the chapter has been written with this in mind, it would be wrong to suggest that this is the only correct way of proceeding. There are good reasons for adopting other patterns, according to the client group, setting, etc. This section describes one or two alternatives (Liebmann 1979: 52–4).

Discussion followed by painting

In this format, much longer is spent on the initial discussion, which is an activity in its own right, rather than just an introduction. This is particularly appropriate for groups which need a long time to get into the artwork; for example, a group of elderly people with mental health difficulties, or a group of long-stay patients on 'rehabilitation wards', or some children's groups. After the discussion has started ideas flowing, the group engages in the artwork. The final discussion tends to be fairly brief, with members of the group mainly showing their pictures to others. (If group members do not have much 'insight', it is pointless to spend a long time on reflective discussion.)

Some groups do not discuss the paintings at the time of the group, but save this for the next session. The format would then be: discussion of last week's images, followed by this week's artwork. Although in general this seems a rather fragmented way of doing things, there can be sound reasons for adopting it. A family therapist using art asked the families he saw to do pictures right at the end of their sessions. That gave him a chance to look at the pictures with a colleague between sessions, so that he could present them positively at the beginning of the next session. These pictures then formed the basis of the discussion, with another theme for a picture being undertaken at the end of the session.

Painting as main activity

For some groups doing the art activity is the main focus and discussion is not very relevant. This is true for groups which may find verbal communication difficult, e.g. groups for people with learning disabilities and some children's groups. Here the importance of the artwork is that it provides a much needed vehicle of communication. It can also be a deliberate choice for groups which tend towards over-verbalisation.

Emphasis on social aspect

This can be important for groups of isolated people who are living in the community, but come together for weekly art sessions in a day hospital or day centre. They may be groups of people with learning disabilities, people with ongoing mental health needs or elderly people. In these groups, talking tends to be encouraged and art activities and themes chosen to facilitate this. Breaks for tea and coffee are also part of the routine.

Another way in which the social aspect can be emphasised is the way preparations are handled. For instance, in a day centre which fosters a self-help ethos members take part in the preparations of the room and take pride in being included in this.

It is up to the therapist or facilitator to develop the most appropriate pattern for their particular group and group members themselves may suggest alternatives. Variations over a period of time may take place, or the group may just wish to 'ring the changes' for one particular session.

Introductions and 'warming up'

Introductions

The main aim of the initial phase of a group session is to bring people together, help them to 'arrive' and to relax before they plunge into an experience that may be new, difficult or strenuous. You can do a lot to encourage a good atmosphere just by the welcome you give to the group members, whether they have arrived from afar or are resident in the institution where the session takes place. If people have travelled some distance, a good way to start can be by having hot drinks available. This also helps to smooth over the awkward period at the beginning when not everyone has arrived and it is inappropriate to make a start.

If people do not already know each other, it is essential to spend some time on introductions. As well as names, it helps to ask for a small piece of introductory information, for example, why people have come, what they are hoping to get from the session(s), or a bit of personal information. Sometimes it is a good idea to structure this and ask for, say, people's hobbies, to avoid the stereotyped responses and 'pigeon-holing' by work labels (as well as the awkwardness for those without jobs). The aim of this time is for people to get to know each other a little, so that they feel more comfortable working together. It can also help you, as facilitator, to get a feel for the people in the group and their interest in it, and this can be helpful in running the sessions.

If a session is one of a series, it may still be necessary to introduce any newcomers and explain to them what the group is about. It is important to check how people are feeling and what is on their minds, especially if the group takes place in an institution. Expressing some of these thoughts and feelings can sometimes help people to 'arrive' mentally and can also provide possible pointers for a theme for the session.

In this introductory session you also need to spell out any ground rules or get the group to agree on certain points, e.g. smoking, timing, breaks, toilets, participation, talking, etc. (see Group Boundaries and Ground Rules section in this chapter). You will also need to explain the nature of the group, what art therapy is or the personal nature of this art group. Some of the phrases that can be useful are:

- not about producing beautiful works of art
- painting as we did when we were children – spontaneously
- exploring in an open-ended way
- no 'right' way of doing it
- expressing our feelings using art materials
- using art in a personal way
- no special ability or disability
- complete statements and finished images are not looked for – scribbles and marks are fine
- relax and use the media in whatever way you want
- no one will be judging the artwork with marks out of ten
- therapists/facilitators will not be making snap interpretations of your work.

Obviously, not all of these remarks are suitable for all groups and you will need to choose and adapt what you say to your group.

Probably a word or two about the materials available will be a good idea, especially if some of the group members have not used them before, or for a long time. The more relaxed people are about using the materials, the more freely and spontaneously they will be able to use them.

'Warm-up' activities

This can be a physical activity or some introductory artwork. Physical 'warm-up' activities include such things as shoulder rubs, milling round and shaking hands, circle dances, etc., which help to get energy flowing. There is a short list of these in Part II, Section A of this book. If you are interested in developing their use further, there are some books listed in the Resources section at the end of the book.

Painting 'warm-up' activities include such things as: passing a piece of paper around for everyone to make a mark; a quick drawing of what is on people's minds; introducing oneself in a picture. There is a list of suggestions in Part II, Section A, and many themes can be adapted for use as 'warm-ups'. The drawings or paintings done at this stage are usually discussed briefly before moving on to the main theme of the session.

In an established group, introductions and 'warm-up' activities may not be needed each time. The group comes together, has a brief discussion about the session's theme and then everyone gets straight on with the artwork. This is possible because the ground rules and way of working have been established and have become an implicit part of the group. If new people join, these ground rules will have to be explained. From time to time, an established group will need to spend some discussion time to reassess its way of working and its ground rules, and possibly to agree on some change if it seems appropriate.

Choosing a theme

There are rather different considerations for groups that meet regularly and for single-occasion groups.

Groups meeting regularly

To start the group, a fairly general theme is needed, to help people to get to know each other and their concerns. Possible starting themes might be:

- Getting to know the media, playing with paint, possibly using wet paper and developing something from it (Part II, Section B, no. 53)
- Any activity from the Media Exploration section (Part II, Section B)
- Introductions (Part II, Section E, no. 125)
- Lifeline (Part II, Section E, no. 140)
- How you are feeling, current preoccupations.

These are just a few ideas. The main thing is to get people started and to be sensitive to their needs. There are several ways of trying to work out how to choose an appropriate theme from one session to the next:

(a) Between sessions, work out what would follow on best and devise an appropriate theme. For example, in a psychiatric hospital acute ward, at the end of one session the discussion was about loneliness. The art therapist worked out a series on friendship (Part II, Section E, no. 173).

(b) Where the art therapy session is part of an overall programme, there may be pointers from other sessions. For example, in a day hospital using art therapy, psychodrama, yoga, psychotherapy and discussion, the art therapy session took place the day after the psychodrama session. The staff team met between the sessions to work out suitable themes for the art session, based on what had emerged from the psychodrama session.

(c) Look at the paintings from the previous session (usually the previous week) with the group to see whether people have any fresh thoughts on them. See what theme emerges from this discussion.

(d) If a particular problem in group relationships seems to be impeding the group's progress, a group painting can often show this up, so that it can be discussed. For example, in a day hospital group, one particular man hid behind his paintings. A group painting showed his contribution squeezed into a corner, demonstrating to the whole group how 'marginalised' he felt.

(e) If a change of direction seems to be required, think through what is needed and select an appropriate theme.

In most of the options so far, the therapist or facilitator takes a large measure of responsibility for choosing the theme, and this can be appropriate, although it does mean that the choice is very much influenced by the therapist's view of members' needs. Where there is a thread of continuity, the group also has a feeling of making progress, step by step, and this can be encouraging. However, the disadvantage of these options is that they are not able to take account of the more immediate feelings and moods of the group. The following options show how these can be included:

(f) The warm-up session or introductory 'round of feelings' can lead to a choice of theme. For example, in one group of young adults there were a lot of feelings about parents, so the facilitator suggested a theme on family life. Possibilities could be:

- how I see myself fitting into family life
- what I got from my Mum and my Dad
- likes and dislikes about my family
- the family set-up in diagram form.

In a group of patients with eating disorders, the initial discussion sometimes gave rise to a theme which the group decided to pursue. Over a period, themes that emerged in this way included feeling stuck, moving forward, letting go of anorexia, 'Where I am now', body image and self-harm (Miles 2002).

(g) Sometimes there is an 'atmosphere' which is intangible but real, especially if the group takes place in an institution or organisation where group members spend a lot of time together. It may be a matter of intuition to pick up these feelings and suggest an appropriate theme. For instance, when I arrived for a weekly session at a women's group at a day centre on a deprived housing estate, I felt an unusual atmosphere of hostility; and no one would talk or felt like doing any artwork. I suggested a theme of 'a safe place' and this enabled the women to start. Afterwards the centre coordinator told me they had been feeling very unsafe because a centre member had breached confidentiality. The theme had helped to unlock their feelings so that the women could begin to discuss the matter.

(h) The 'round of feelings' could be based on what people felt after the previous week's session, and this could lead to the next theme, as above.

(i) If the facilitator usually introduces a theme without a 'round of feelings', it can be good to have a choice of themes so that the group can choose.

(j) In peer groups, such as staff training groups, a list can be passed round for people to choose what they want to explore.

(k) Some groups come together to explore particular issues or ways of working and then the themes chosen reflect these. See, for instance, Chapter 6, Example 7 (anger management art therapy group) and books such as: Cook and Heales (2001) – themes exploring spirituality; Luzzatto (2000) – themes for cancer patients; Ross (1997) – themes for children in schools; Safran (2002) – themes on AD/HD; Silverstone (1997) – themes on person-centred counselling.

Any theme chosen should be flexible enough for people to interpret in their own way, according to their needs.

Some practical points will need to be borne in mind. Group paintings and murals need preparation, rooms have to be rearranged for group projects, special materials have to be organised. There is no 'right' way of choosing a theme. It is a matter for each facilitator or therapist to work out in the most appropriate way, according to their own preferred style, the needs of the group and the facilities at their disposal.

Single-occasion groups

The choice of theme here depends very much on the aims and goals of the group. Here are some examples of themes chosen (some of these groups are described more fully in Chapter 6, and all the themes are explained in Part II of this book):

1   Residential children's workers attending an in-service training course were asked to start by joining in a group mural. After discussion, this was followed by the theme 'My Family Tree', each person drawing their own family as a tree. This gave rise to discussion of family experiences as seen from a child's point of view.

2   A women's group experiencing difficulties did a group drawing in
    which each person had a different coloured crayon and contributed in
    turn. The resulting patterns of communication were discussed.
3   A group of cancer patients finding it difficult to contemplate the future
    did paintings on the theme of journeys they wanted to make.
4   An introductory day for a church group containing adults and children
    included:

- Introductions – name and a personal interest
- Round Robin drawings (see Part II, Section I, no. 296)
- Conversation in paint, with one partner
- Paint yourself as a kind of food
- Lunch (shared)
- Group story on long sheet of paper, made up of everyone's
  individual stories, interwoven in silence (see Part II, Section H,
  no. 248)
- Writing based on group story
- Group collage.

5   An introductory evening for a group of professionals included:

- How I am feeling
- Conversation in paint, in pairs
- Group painting (no theme).

6   An afternoon for a peace education group included:

- Introduce yourself in a picture
- Painting in pairs
- Group painting on theme of 'What peace means to me'.

In all these examples, plenty of time was allowed for discussion after each
activity and at the end.

Themes in relation to client groups

One might think that using a particular theme would always have the same
outcome. This is hardly ever the case. The following example demonstrates
this. Three different art therapists, commenting on the theme 'Draw an
advertisement for yourself', had very different experiences (Liebmann 1979:
127):

Therapist A: The purpose of this is to look at positive self-image. It is
              useful with a particularly depressed group – lots of positive
              feedback from group members to other individuals.

Therapist B: A difficult theme which needs careful introduction, but can become very negative, I've found.

Therapist C: I usually suggest that people consider not only those aspects of themselves which are worthwhile, but also what kind of people they wish to attract . . . becoming conscious of how one presents oneself publicly is a difficult enterprise, and people often present their disabilities and uncertainties rather than their abilities and good points.

The first two therapists were working with inpatients and day patients in a hospital and the third was working in a social services day centre for clients with mental health difficulties. Another art therapist, working with a variety of groups, summed up his experiences succinctly: 'I have found that the outcome of a session depends less on the theme chosen than on what the clients bring with them to the group.' Thus what actually happens in the group is influenced by many factors such as:

- outside limitations
- the setting in which the group functions
- the particular client group
- the stage the group has reached
- current mood and preoccupations
- the kind of group and its emphasis on certain issues and ways of working
- the style of facilitation
- the choice of a particular theme or activity
- the way discussion is handled.

All these factors will have a bearing on the outcome of any one session. There are some notes on different client groups in Chapter 7. However, the important thing to keep in mind is that you are choosing a theme in relation to your group and its current needs.

Engaging in the artwork

This is the time when everyone is usually totally absorbed in what they are doing. A 'no talking' rule can intensify this experience, which can be very deep. Sometimes it happens naturally, especially with experienced groups. Facilitators should try to ensure that there will not be any interruptions during this period (e.g. latecomers, notices about lunch, etc.), as these can be very unsettling and break the 'spell' of deep concentration. Any time limits should be announced at the beginning.

The actual doing of the artwork is really important. It is not just the time needed to get something on paper, which can be discussed, but a time during which non-verbal processes take over and people are working things out through paint, clay, etc. This process cannot be adequately described in words, and this is why it is important that group facilitators have first-hand experience of doing artwork and trying out particular themes themselves.

There are some groups for whom making artwork can promote useful conversation which is to be encouraged. For instance, some adolescents who are usually too self-conscious to express opinions can 'open up' while they are engaged in a group painting or working with clay. Encouraging conversation can also be important for groups of adults with learning disabilities or elderly people living in the community but attending weekly art therapy sessions. Here talking and making friends are part of the purpose of the sessions.

The beginning of the time for artwork can be awkward for some. There are materials to organise and the facilitator needs to be available to help here. When everyone has got what they need and settled down, there is usually a short hesitant period while people sit and think about what they are going to do. This is fine and should cause no concern. However, occasionally there are one or two people who are really 'stuck'. It can be a terrifying experience to stare at a blank piece of paper while all around everyone else seems to know what they want to do. The therapist or facilitator needs to help out here, perhaps with some gentle questions, to draw out what that person feels about the theme. (It may not be appropriate for them, in some unforeseen way; in which case it should be modified or discarded.) If everyone is stuck, it is probably because the explanation of the theme was not clear enough, or because the introductory period was too rushed. The only thing to do here is to go through it again, perhaps with more group discussion, rather than leave everyone struggling.

People work at very different speeds. Some people rush into things and finish very quickly; others work at a slow and measured pace. This means that people will often finish at different times. Two things can help here: fast workers can be encouraged to do a second painting while waiting, or to reflect in a constructive way on what they have done. Slow workers may not finish (and usually this does not matter), but can be helped by being informed when time is nearly up so that they can decide what is most important. It is sometimes really interesting to watch how people paint, and see where they put the greatest energy, where they are more tentative, where they wait and reflect. If you are not participating in the artwork stage, it can be very worthwhile just to observe what is going on.

If the group is a short session (e.g. a weekly two-hour session), it is often a good idea to clear up the materials at the end of doing the artwork, especially if the discussion has to take place in the same space. However, if the group takes place over a day, weekend or week including several exercises followed by discussion, it is best to leave clearing up until the end of the day.

Discussion

The physical arrangements for the discussion are important. Everybody needs to be able to see what is being discussed. It facilitates group cohesion and interaction if everyone can also have eye contact with one another. Some groups can manage these while staying in the same positions as for the artwork, or by standing round the finished work if it is a group project. Some groups are lucky enough to have a messy painting area and a comfortable relaxation area with armchairs and carpet, so that everyone can sit in a circle with the paintings in the middle on the floor.

Leading a discussion about the paintings produced is another whole group session. There are many models of groupwork available and it is a good idea to consult some of the books listed under Groupwork in the Resources section at the end of this book. It is important that everyone in the group is clear about the process of discussion that is being used. I will outline three of the most usual models used with personal art or art therapy groups: everyone takes turns; focus on one or two pictures; focus on group dynamics.

Everyone takes turns

This is the most usual way of sharing the results of the session and can be very fruitful. It is essential to say whether everyone is expected to share their paintings, or whether there is no obligation. The therapist or facilitator may ask if anyone would like to start, and everyone else follows on round the circle in turn; or the first person can choose the next one, and so on; or everyone takes a turn when it feels right. If there is time left at the end, a general discussion may develop.

If the group is large, sharing all the paintings takes a long time and it is important to allow for this. If time runs out before one or two members have shared their work there may be an 'unfinished' feel about the session for them. The facilitator needs to decide, in conjunction with the group, how much time each person has, and the method of timekeeping. Sometimes not all members of the group want equal time and the timing sorts itself out; at other times a formal five minutes each is needed.

The facilitator can encourage group participation by asking what other people think, so that not all comments are directed just to her or him. If the facilitator has taken part in the artwork, then she/he will probably be expected to share too, unless time runs out. Here the facilitator or therapist treads a fine line between being and not being a member of the group – disclosing something of themselves, yet not burdening the group with their most pressing problems. There are several advantages in taking turns:

(a) For people who have not done it before, talking about their paintings (which may contain very personal statements) can be an exposing experience. When everyone takes a turn, people feel they are not alone and that 'breaking the ice' is a group endeavour. (However, it is wise to respect group members who do not wish to share their paintings, for whatever reason.)

(b) In a new group, everyone sharing can help group members to get to know each other through their pictures.

(c) In an ongoing group, the security of structured sharing can help people to build up trust and become more adventurous about what they are willing to disclose in their paintings and the discussion.

(d) It is a way of ensuring that quieter members of the group have their share of time and that certain members of the group do not dominate the discussion.

(e) The 'equal shares' aspect of this method appeals to many peer and self-help groups.

There are, however, some disadvantages:

(a) Each person will only have a fairly short time (unless the group is very small), and this can be frustrating. Sharing in pairs or subgroups can help here.

(b) The discussion usually sticks fairly closely to the pictures, and sometimes this can be superficial.

(c) Structuring the discussion can be seen as artificial in that it removes some of the free flow of group interaction. The safety of the structure is seen as an obstacle to exploring conflicts which may arise.

Focus on one or two pictures

Some therapists and facilitators feel that taking turns is artificial and leads to superficiality. They feel more is gained by exploring one or two members' issues more than the rest, or using the whole discussion time on one or two pictures. The individuals may be chosen, or choose themselves, because their need is greatest at that moment. Others can then be included by asking if they have had any similar experiences. Sometimes the sharing of just one painting can lead to a deep discussion which involves everyone in the group in a very meaningful way.

Focus on group dynamics

In this kind of discussion the group is simply available for anything to happen. The result may be a general discussion, or under the guidance of a skilled therapist a verbal psychotherapy group based loosely on the paintings. The therapist may ask if anyone would like to talk about their

pictures and then wait to see what comes up. In a free-ranging psychotherapy group, expression of real feelings and conflicts is encouraged. For
instance, if a group member gets angry this may be looked at in terms of
projections of feelings about that member's parents or spouse. In this way it
is hoped to resolve conflicts felt by group members, and which may have
brought them into therapy. Members of the group are encouraged to help
each other and pool their experiences. In this model of discussion, the
pictures are the jumping-off point. They may play a large part in the
discussion or have a relatively minor role, and rarely will there be time to
look at all the paintings in depth.

Therapists leading such groups need considerable experience, which may
be gained through training or by co-facilitating a similar group with
someone experienced. It is worth adding that there is hardly ever enough
time to process all the material that comes up and therapists and facilitators
will have to help the group to cope with this (Skaife and Huet 1998; Waller
1993).

Interpretation

In this area there are one or two assumptions people may make, which can
be quite misleading. This does not happen so much now, as art therapy has
become much more widely known, but it is important to be aware of them.
The first assumption is that it is the therapist's job to interpret group
members' paintings. This assumption has its origin in one of the first uses of
art therapy, as an adjunct to psychoanalysis. Patients produced pictures as
material for the analysis, in the same way as dream material might be
explored using the same theoretical framework (e.g. Freudian, Jungian,
Kleinian, etc.). The process of painting them was not seen as important.
This kind of interpretation always takes place in a particular theoretical
framework (or psychoanalytical school) and requires considerable training
and experience. Art therapy groups of this kind are led by art therapists
qualified and experienced in these particular frameworks.

However, most facilitators and therapists find themselves working with
groups in institutions which have no single therapeutic stance; or with
teams with a medical orientation emphasising medication rather than
psychological treatments; or with community organisations which do not
operate within a therapeutic framework. It is up to facilitators and therapists to choose for themselves the theories they find most helpful, which
can range from several psychodynamically oriented theories to the many
humanistic perspectives.

The second widely held assumption is that interpretation is based on a
knowledge of symbols in a one-to-one equivalence of meaning. This is
rarely the case. More usually, symbols have a range of culturally based
meanings (e.g. the sun can indicate summer, light, warmth, heat). Most

symbols also have a subjective meaning, which can vary from person to person, usually within the range of accepted meanings, but sometimes completely outside it, according to that person's experience.

Working in similar contexts may give rise to symbols with a range of similar meanings, but care is needed to avoid extrapolating too easily from one context to another. For instance, an art therapist in a psychiatric hospital, working with many depressed patients, may notice several black and red paintings. If she/he then sees another black and red painting, perhaps elsewhere, she/he may or may not be correct in guessing that the painter is depressed. There is the apocryphal story of the man who painted a black and red picture and then announced that it showed his relief that his bank account was 'in the black' once more. Obviously the wider experience a therapist or facilitator has, the more their guesses are likely to be near the mark.

At one level we are all engaged in interpretations. We all look at the world in different ways and with different assumptions about it. This often means that our interpretations of an event or picture say as much about us and our frames of reference as they do about the matter in hand. (In Part II some good exercises to explore this are Section I, nos. 288–91.) While our interpretations might be true for ourselves, we must beware of foisting them on other people.

There is a sense in which a painting can sometimes 'speak back' to the artist. This is a process to encourage as it enables people to have a dialogue with themselves. People sometimes need to sit with their paintings for a little while to let this happen.

Interpretation is obviously a minefield where facilitators can make many mistakes. Are there any guidelines? The most important thing is how the painter of the picture sees it and what he/she meant. In an ongoing group, as trust is built up and people feel safe, they will be prepared to be more open and disclose more information and feelings.

A sensitive facilitator or therapist and perceptive group members can also help someone to draw out 'hidden depths' for themselves, but this needs to be suggested rather than presented as fact. A particular interpretation may be more to do with the speaker than the painter, or the painter of the picture may not be ready to hear what is being suggested. There has to be a tentativeness about any interpretation and an acceptance on the part of the recipient. One way of being sensitive to other people's artwork is to own our views of their pictures. So group members can be encouraged to ask questions such as 'Could you say what that corner bit is about?' or 'To me that bit looks like . . .' or 'When I look at your picture, I am reminded of . . .'.

In an ongoing group a woman did a detailed drawing of cracking ice to demonstrate how she had felt when her marriage was cracking up. Several months later, the art therapist was leading a one-day workshop in another town, and commented about a jagged painted pattern, 'The last time I saw a pattern a bit like that, it was about someone's marriage breaking up.' She was fairly amazed to receive the reply, 'Well, you've guessed right first time, I'm going through it at the moment.' This sort of interpretation is intuitive guesswork, based on experience of others and of oneself and on a familiarity with visual communication. To summarise, I have listed below some of the possible ways of looking at the group's pictures:

1   Each person talks about his or her work, without comment or questions from others.
2   In addition to (1), other people ask questions and make comments. This needs to be done sensitively. If a comment is not accepted by the painter, it may be because she/he is not ready for it, or because the comment is inappropriate. In either case, it would be unwise to take it any further.
3   People reflect and see if their paintings 'speak back' to them.
4   Artwork review. It can be rewarding to look back at pictures done over a period of time to see if there are any patterns or recurring themes. Sometimes people can see pictures they did some time ago in a fresh light, and this can bring new realisations.
5   Gestalt technique. This can be used with any art product. The painter is encouraged to talk about the picture in the first person and to become each part of the painting in turn. The assumption behind this is that different parts of the painting may represent different sides of someone's personality. For instance: 'I am this tree. I'm quite a strong tree, and I'm well rooted, but I don't seem to have many leaves. It's winter and I'm cold and bare.' After this, the speaker may reflect on whether this rings true for him or her in a wider way. After becoming each part in turn, one can go on to create a dialogue between the different parts of the painting representing different sides of a person. This technique can be very powerful so is best used in a small or established group where there is a lot of trust and support available for group members.

Ending the session

Many sessions are bound by institutional timetables, and it is vital to finish on time. Sometimes the clatter of plates nearby is a cogent signal. It is good to try to end the session on a positive note, perhaps with a comment that sums up the session or thanks to people for coming, etc. Some facilitators and therapists like to include an ending ritual or exercise.

On a whole-day or weekend workshop, one way of closing is to have a round of comments on, say, 'What I got out of the day/weekend' or 'One thing I enjoyed/will remember about the day/weekend', etc. Often there is an evaluation form to fill in. Rather than finishing with this, it feels better to timetable this for just before the end of the session/workshop and then finish with a final round or ritual. Whatever the situation, the ending of the session should bring people back to the here and now so that they can carry on with normal life. Facilitators and therapists should try to make sure that no one leaves the group with any problems or worries which will prevent them from carrying on their day-to-day lives.

Care taken in the introduction of the session (see earlier section of this chapter) will avoid trails of 'unfinished business', but occasionally there will be one or two problems of this nature and the facilitator has to try to deal with them. In institutions there are usually plenty of back-up facilities in the form of other staff and clients to talk to, or the therapist can see a person who is upset afterwards. In community groups this is not so easy. The facilitator can provide information on other opportunities to continue working on the same lines, but it is wiser to try to keep the group experience at a level that is easy for everyone to cope with.

Finally, there is the clearing up. Sometimes the situation dictates that the facilitator is left with this, but often helping to clear up can be a practical way for people to wind down and get back to ordinary life. If everyone joins in, it is also an expression of group cohesion and gives a good feel to the end of the session. Even if much of the clearing up has been done after the artwork, there are usually paintings and drawings to put away, cups to be washed or equipment to be stacked.

Group process over time

This section will not discuss group process in detail as there are many books (some listed in Resources section) on groupwork which deal with this in depth. It is worth reading one or two of these to clarify your thinking about your group.

In a series of sessions that comes to a definite end, there is a progression of stages that most groups go through. These can be described in various ways from a simple three-stage process such as beginning, middle and end to more sophisticated models (sometimes including as many as nine stages) taking into account many facets of the group. In a theme-based personal art or art therapy group which meets regularly, I have found the following stages useful in describing group development over time:

1   *Beginning*: the group meets and starts its activity. It is probably very dependent on the leader to initiate everything at this stage.
2   *Finding its feet*: the group gets used to the way of working and mis-understandings are cleared up. If it is an open group some people leave, discovering this activity is not for them, or it is not what they thought it was. Others become more committed.

3   *Group cohesion*: people come knowing what to expect and looking forward to group sessions. Trust is built up.
4   *Disclosure*: group members become more willing to disclose themselves in their paintings and in the discussion. At this stage there is often a very deep sharing as people openly grapple with some of their most pressing problems.
5   *Ending*: this is often accompanied by a variety of feelings such as depression, confusion, anger and relief, even if it is only a temporary break. If it is the end of the group, there is also the question of 'What next?'

An art therapy group has these stages in common with other groups and it is good to be aware of them and prepared to meet them. These stages are not completely separate – they often overlap each other. To a certain extent they are also present in a single-occasion group such as a day or weekend workshop.

Some groups do not have a definite ending. They continue to meet, ideally on the level of stage 4 of deep sharing through painting and other artwork. Many groups like this have a membership which changes over time. Then each member who joins usually goes through these stages individually, helped by more experienced group members at each stage. Joining and leaving can be big issues. If too many people join or leave at the same time the nature of the group can change quite radically. If a group is functioning well, it is probably best for people to join in ones and twos, so that the ethos of the group is maintained and can be extended to include newcomers. Similarly, people leaving a group can affect the group significantly, especially if those remaining feel abandoned or left behind.

For a time-boundaried series (e.g. ten sessions), there is often an evaluation questionnaire to fill in and sometimes some form of outcome measurement. It is important to think about the best place for these. So, for instance, an evaluation of the group as an experience might best be done just before the end, while feelings of being in the group are accessible. An outcome measurement might be done a week or two later, when people are clearer about what they have gained from the group. Post-group interviews can be helpful for this and also for helping people to work out their next steps, or facilitating a handover to another professional.

Recording and evaluation

A group session is not finished (from the therapist or facilitator's point of view) until whatever recording system is in place has been completed. This should be done as soon as possible after the group. Any discussions with other staff or planning for the next session should also be done as soon as possible, or at least timetabled. Any contributions to evaluation need to be undertaken. Recording and evaluation have developed into large topics, so they are the subject of the next chapter.

References

Barber, V. and Campbell, J. (1999) 'Living colour in art therapy: visual and verbal narrative of black and white', in J. Campbell, M. Liebmann, F. Brooks, J. Jones and C. Ward (eds) *Art Therapy, Race and Culture*, London: Jessica Kingsley Publishers.

Benson, J. (2001) *Working More Creatively with Groups*, 2nd edn, London: Routledge.

Brown, A. (1992) *Groupwork*, 3rd edn, Aldershot: Ashgate.

Campbell, J. (1993) *Creative Art in Groupwork*, Bicester: Speechmark.

Case, C. and Dalley, T. (1992) *The Handbook of Art Therapy*, London: Tavistock/ Routledge.

Cook, C. and Heales, B. C. (2001) *Seeding the Spirit: The Appleseed Workbook*, Birmingham: Woodbrooke Quaker Study Centre.

Disability Rights Commission (DRC) (2002) *Making Access to Goods and Services Easier for Disabled Customers: A Practical Guide for Small Businesses and other Small Service Providers*, Stratford: DRC.

Greenwood, H. and Layton, G. (1987) 'An out patient art therapy group', *Inscape*, summer: 12–19.

Greenwood, H. and Layton, G. (1991) 'Taking the piss', *Inscape*, winter: 7–14.

Liebmann, M. F. (1979) 'A study of structured art therapy groups', unpublished MA thesis, Birmingham Polytechnic.

Luzzatto, P. (2000) 'The creative journey: a model for short-term group art therapy with posttreatment cancer patients', *Art Therapy: Journal of the American Art Therapy Association*, 17, 4: 265–9.

Miles, M. (2002) 'Eating disorder patients: working with an emerging theme', personal communication.

Ross, C. (1997) *Something to Draw On: Activities and Interventions Using an Art Therapy Approach*, London: Jessica Kingsley Publishers.

Safran, D. S. (2002) *Art Therapy and AD/HD: Diagnostic and Therapeutic Approaches*, London: Jessica Kingsley Publishers.

Silverstone, L. (1997) *Art Therapy: The Person-Centred Way*, 2nd edn, London: Jessica Kingsley Publishers.

Skaife, S. and Huet, V. (1998) 'Introduction', in S. Skaife and V. Huet (eds) *Art Psychotherapy Groups*, London: Routledge.

Waller, D. (1993) *Group Interactive Art Therapy: Its Use in Training and Treatment*, London: Routledge.

Whitaker, D. S. (2001) *Using Groups to Help People*, 2nd edn, London: Brunner-Routledge.

Chapter 3

Recording, evaluation and evidence-based practice

It is not easy to record or evaluate such a fluid experience as a group art or art therapy session, but you need to make some attempt at it in order to make progress. Recording and evaluation can be approached in several ways and some of them are outlined in this chapter. These processes, together with audit and evidence-based practice, are assuming a greater importance in many spheres. However, detailed discussion is beyond the scope of this book, so this chapter will mention them briefly and refer readers to the burgeoning literature on these topics for further investigation.

There are several reasons for the interest in these areas. One is the need to know that we are doing the best we can for our clients. Another is the need to apply limited resources in the most cost-effective way. Also important is the need for therapists and facilitators to continue learning and improve their practice. In the NHS, the *National Service Framework for Mental Health* (1999a) and *Clinical Governance: Quality in the new NHS* (1999b) give guidance on good practice. Other organisations and institutions are following suit. It is important to choose the best methods of recording and evaluation for your purpose. Often several methods can be used together.

Recording

Any evaluation must rest on some kind of information gathered, whether this is done formally or informally, as an overview or in detail. Here are some things you might think of recording and methods of doing so.

Basic information about the group sessions

Wherever you are working, you will need to keep some sort of record of the group, as detailed as you have time for and appropriate to the setting in which you work. Write down such things as:

- basic information: date, venue, number of session, clientele, members and therapists/facilitators present/absent

- aims for session
- theme or activity used
- how the group went: what actually happened
- how the group felt: initial mood, emotional graph of the group, facilitator's or therapist's feelings, levels of interaction and disclosure, etc.
- individuals: what artwork they produced, how they reacted to discussion of it
- facilitator(s)/therapist(s): what you did; co-facilitators or therapists (if any); any students/trainees present and their roles; how you related to others
- summary and future plans.

Clinical notes

If you are working in an organisation or institution with a therapeutic orientation such as a hospital or day centre, you will also have to write clinical notes. These are notes kept on individuals' work and progress, according to the format of the institution. It is good practice to complete the notes immediately, preferably with both facilitators contributing if they have both been involved in the running of the group. Clients should be told that records are being kept. Most institutions now have open records policies, so clients will have access to the clinical notes you write about them. In some places there is provision for clients to add to their own clinical notes. This means it is important to avoid value judgements and interpretations as far as possible. If they need to be included, make it clear that it is your opinion and not a 'fact'. Clinical notes should be kept in a secure and locked cabinet, to be accessed only by the therapists and members of the clinical team.

Artwork produced

If you are working in the community, people may want to take their artworks home. If not, you will need somewhere to store them securely and confidentially – especially if the room where you work has multiple uses. If you are working in a therapeutic institution, you may be expected to keep all the artwork as records, at least for the duration of the group. This is useful for picture reviews with clients and for supervision or case reports. Let members of the group know that the artworks are theirs to take away at the end of the group. It is a good idea to jot down any comments made by the artist about their artwork (or better still get the artist to do so). Ask everyone to write the date on their work. If artwork is likely to crumble or decay or is to be taken home, a photographic record is useful. Polaroid cameras are useful in providing quick results, such as giving children copies to take away with them. Clinical notes should contain a description of any artwork and/or a small sketch of it.

Photography and video can also be used to record artworks. Digital cameras can be particularly useful in charting the visual development of artwork and video can pick up nuances of group dynamics in a unique way. But both these methods are intrusive and may alter the whole process, so they need to be thought about carefully. Group members' permission is also needed, as it is if clients' artworks are used for other purposes, e.g. talks. This permission should be in writing if the pictures are to be published in any permanent format.

Process recording

This is an attempt to write down as much detail as possible about a session, including all your thoughts and feelings, and is quite time consuming. It needs to be done as soon as possible after the session. Its advantage is that it can help to make connections between seemingly unrelated events of the session. It is probably a method to be used occasionally, perhaps as preparation for a supervision session. It is not appropriate for this kind of recording to be included in clinical notes.

Checklist for each participant

This method is useful for being consistent in recording the same information about each participant. You need to prepare a checklist with headings on it (e.g. name, materials used, body language, interactions, image produced, mood, etc.). Photocopy it and fill in one for each participant immediately after the group (Case and Dalley 1992: 162–3).

Group therapy interaction chronogram

This is a useful method of charting the interactions of members at different phases of the group, based on work by Murray Cox (1988) and developed for an art therapy context by Caroline Case and Tessa Dalley (1992). Each group participant (including the therapist) is represented by a circle divided into three sections (see Figure 3.1). In section 1 are written that person's actions during the first quarter of the session, in section 2 the next half of the session and in section 3 the final quarter. The circles are arranged in the order of seating in the group, and arrows can be drawn to show interactions. If you want to use this method, read the section in *The Handbook of Art Therapy* (Case and Dalley 1992: 163–7).

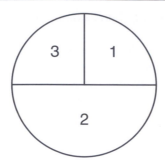

Figure 3.1 Group therapy interaction chronogram for one participant

Group book

It can be useful to have a group book available for comments. This can sometimes pick up feelings that members have not expressed in the session, for a variety of reasons. The book (with a heading for the day's session) and pen need to be left in a convenient place where participants can write in it without being conspicuous.

Evaluation with co-facilitators and other staff

It is vital to set aside time to reflect on the group session, both to learn from it and to plan for the next session, which may need to pick up on issues which have come up. There may also be issues to pass on to other staff if the group takes place in a hospital or day centre. It is important to let group members know the ways that you will be doing this, e.g. notes to key workers, supervision, etc. Here are some ways of doing this.

After each session

One of the advantages of a co-facilitator is that there are two of you to discuss what happened. This can help you to stand back and see the group in perspective and is a good opportunity to check your thinking. If you are running a group on your own, it is very useful to find another appropriate person to talk to. Sometimes a short reflection time is useful and facilitators may want to do an image of how they perceived the session to aid discussion. Below are a few suggestions of questions to ask to help evaluate your group:

• Were any of these positive qualities present: good feelings, enjoyment, commitment, courage, energy, co-operation, sharing?

- Were there any negative feelings, and if so were they adequately dealt with?
- Was there any unfinished business, and if so how could it be dealt with?
- How did the co-facilitators work together?
- What did group members get out of it?
- Do they/you want to continue working in this way?
- Looking back at the session(s), was the end result of the experience rewarding and growth promoting? (This may take a little while to judge.)
- Were the aims of the session(s) achieved?

This is also a good opportunity to record the group session in whatever way you have chosen to do.

Review of several sessions or whole group

It is useful to review how a group is going over a period of time, or when it has ended. This may bring to light significant issues such as group development, drop-out rate, progress of members. More details of this kind of review can be found in *Using Groups to Help People* (Whitaker 2001: Chapter 18). Sometimes this kind of review is included in supervision.

Supervision

This is vital to continued learning and development. It is important to distinguish between management supervision and clinical supervision. Management supervision is usually concerned with the place of a group in the overall function of an agency and such things as caseloads, boundaries, health and safety, etc. Clinical supervision is concerned with what happens in the group itself and the roles and functioning of the therapists. It is usually undertaken by a separate person, either a designated and appropriately experienced clinical supervisor within the agency or an external supervisor. In the UK your regional group of the British Association of Art Therapists may be able to help here, or you can consult the BAAT lists of approved supervisors and private practitioners. In other countries, consult your art therapy association (there are some addresses in the Resources section). If there are few experienced people in your area, a peer consultation group will be the next best, so that people working in similar ways can learn from each other.

Whatever the framework, the task is to learn to improve relevant skills by discussion of work in progress with more experienced therapists and facilitators. The content of these sessions can be quite diverse: group dynamics, warming-up techniques, coping with institutions, presenting case material, and so on. On a more informal level, it is good to get together with others working in similar ways, just to share approaches, thoughts and views.

If you are using art with groups in a personal way on your own, you may be able to get support from your local or regional art therapists. In most areas there are formal and informal occasions for art therapists to meet and exchange their ways of working. Contact the British Association of Art Therapists (see Resources section for address) for details of your regional group coordinator or to consult the list of supervisors.

Feedback to other staff

If you work in an institution where the art or art therapy group is part of an overall programme, it is vital to give feedback to other staff; e.g. nurses on wards, community psychiatric nurses, doctors in charge of treatment, social workers, teachers, care co-ordinators, etc. Sometimes this entails notes to key workers or a brief verbal report in a staff meeting. Sometimes there is the opportunity of going through the pictures to explain what people have experienced and communicated. This can facilitate a broader understanding of people's problems. For instance, an elderly lady attending a day hospital for depression painted a picture of her sister who had died. Other staff were previously unaware of this, as she had never spoken about her sister. It is important to let group members know of any regular methods you are using and if you have fed back any particular concerns.

Evaluation involving group members

Group feedback on each session

A big sheet of paper can be posted on the wall with three columns: Liked, Disliked and Bright Ideas – or a pictorial version with a 'smiley face' 'frowny face' and a lightbulb or candle. Members of the group call out anything that comes to mind, from 'I liked using the paints', 'The chairs are hard' to 'Can we have tea at the beginning instead of the end?' The whole process only takes five minutes and can give some pointers about general reactions and points to bear in mind for the next session. However, it will rarely include everyone's views. This method can also be used as a way of reviewing several sessions to see if a group is meeting members' needs. A children's version of instant feedback can be something physical such as: 'Clap your hands if you really enjoyed the session. Stay standing if it was OK. Sit down if you didn't enjoy it at all.' A method for adolescents might be to ask them at the beginning of the session to write their expectations/ hopes on a post-it note. At the end of the session everyone sticks them anonymously on a sheet headed 'Expectations met/not met'.

Individual feedback sheet for each session

This is a way of getting everyone's views, but can be time consuming for both group members and therapists/facilitators. Questions should concentrate on group process for members, e.g. how people felt about the session, how relevant it was to their needs, etc. Sometimes an evaluation form can be very short, with just three questions on it, e.g. best and worst things about the session, and maybe a list of 'feeling' words for people to circle such as happy, sad, bored, enjoyed it, angry, frustrated, inspired, and so on. This was used successfully for a short-life group for homeless people in a hostel where there was a high turnover of members. You may need to be sensitive to those with literacy problems. Children may find it easier to choose from a series of faces with different expressions. Sometimes it may be appropriate to ask for feedback from people connected with group members, e.g. parents/carers, social workers. This needs to be discussed with group members.

Individual feedback on whole group

In a community or short-term group this is probably best handled by including an evaluation session or questionnaire at the end of the sessions. This should focus on members' views about aspects of the group and the way it was run. Sometimes it is useful to include some five-point or ten-point scales, either numerically or in words (e.g. very much/quite a lot/a bit/ not much/not at all) or a visual analogue scale (a 10 cm line with 'worst' at one end and 'best' at the other – this reduces the focus on numbers but can be measured by a ruler afterwards). Again, bear in mind group members with literacy or language problems. Questions can be pared down to a minimum, translated or handled verbally (see, for instance, Chapter 6, Example 14, Asian Women's Group). Parents and carers can help children to fill in simple questionnaires. Examples of questions can be:

- How much did you enjoy the group? (five- or ten-point scale)
- How much benefit/learning did you get? (five- or ten-point scale)
- What did you like best/least overall?
- Did any sessions stand out as particularly meaningful?
- Were any sessions of little value?
- Was there anything you would have liked to be different?
- Any other comments?

It is often difficult to get questionnaires returned. If this is likely to be the case, include them as part of the last session.

Picture review

In an ongoing group in a therapeutic institution there may be more emphasis on progress of individuals. If this is the case, it can be useful to spend a group session in which each person reflects on their work over a period of time – say, every four to eight weeks – to chart changes and progress and formulate future needs.

Personal progress/outcomes

In some institutions the clients contribute to their clinical notes. This depends on the institution's and therapist's style of record keeping. For formal therapy groups, as well as inviting clients to an interview beforehand (see Chapter 2, Setting Up the Group), it is good to ask what they are hoping to get out of the group. Then, at the end of the group, they can be asked how far they have achieved what they were hoping for, and also whether there were other (sometimes unexpected) gains or developments. This can be done by questionnaire, interview or both.

One way I have done this is to give prospective participants a sheet to write down a list of the problems bringing them to the group. For each problem they tick a position on a verbal five-point scale as to how bad this problem is (terrible/very bad/quite bad/bit of a problem/not a problem). They repeat the process at the end of the group sessions and often find that their perception of their problems has shifted. There are also spaces for people to write down their goals (or what they are hoping for) and the changes they want to make. Solution focused brief therapy scaling questions can be useful here. Before the group, help members to be clear about their preferred future, i.e. when the problem is solved. Then ask them:

- Where do you place yourself, on a scale of 0 to 10, in relation to where you want to be?
- Where would you like to be at the end of the group, on a scale of 0 to 10?

At the end of the group, ask them:

- Where are you now, on a scale of 0 to 10?

This can be used as a measurable evaluation of the effectiveness of a series of sessions (George et al. 1999: 16, 31).

Some arts therapy departments organise their whole referral process around clients setting goals and then evaluating how far they have reached them (CESU 1997; Manners 1998).

Measuring outcomes

There are many standardised questionnaires that can be used for this which have been validated across large numbers of people. Participants are asked to fill them in at the beginning and end of a series of sessions and the differences in scores give an indication of the outcomes of the group. Therapists and facilitators need to share with clients the purpose of any measures used and what will happen with responses to the questionnaires. They also need to follow up on any promises made, e.g. to share the results. It is important to choose a measure which is:

- valid, that is, it measures the changes you want: for instance, it is not very useful to use a questionnaire designed to measure depression for a group of people whose problems are connected with anger
- feasible to use – easy for clients to fill in, easy to score, cheap to buy and relevant to your group
- reliable and consistent (Sharry 2001: 109).

Examples of commonly used measures are:

1   CORE (Clinical Outcomes in Routine Evaluation), which includes 34 items rating well-being, symptoms, life functioning and risk behaviours (Barkham and Mellor-Clark 2000: 137). Details of CORE IMS (CORE Information Management System) can be found in the Resources section.
2   OQ-45 (Outcome Questionnaire), which includes 45 items rating symptomatic distress, social and interpersonal functioning (Sharry 2001: 109). Contact details are in the Resources section.
3   Avon Mental Health Measure (South West MIND 1996), aimed at helping service users to assess their functioning and needs, to help decide what services they need. It includes tables on physical, social, behaviour, access and mental health aspects.
4   There are lists of measures in several books, such as *Essentials of Outcome Measurement* (Ogles *et al.* 2002) and *Measuring Health: Guide to Rating Scales and Questionnaires* (McDowell and Newell 1996). Research and development support departments can often help and advise in this area.

Visual outcomes

Many therapists, facilitators and their clients notice changes in clients' artwork as they make progress. There is a considerable body of case study evidence of such changes – greater use of colour, more imaginative use of materials and space, more detail, different shapes, greater involvement in the process, to name but a few. However, there is so far (to my knowledge) no robust, validated visual art therapy outcome measure, though several art therapists are working on ways to remove subjectivity in this area (e.g. Corcos 2002; Lewis and Williams 2002).

An interesting book exploring different ways of measuring visual elements is *Formal Elements Art Therapy Scale Manual* (Gantt and Tabone 1998). It includes visual elements such as use of colour, how much of the paper is used, etc.

Audit

Audit is a process that assesses practice against a predefined standard. It asks the questions 'Has the right thing been done?' and 'Has it been done right?' (Parry 1996; Wood 1999: 56), also 'What are we doing, with whom?' The audit process or cycle can be seen as having four steps:

1   Defining standards for clinical care.
2   Comparing actual practice with these standards.
3   Implementing change to bring practice up to standard.
4   Repeating the cycle at appropriate intervals (Healy 1998: 32). This is important to measure change over a period of time.

One of the important things to audit is equal opportunities monitoring. So, for instance, some years ago, I noticed that I had few referrals from other professionals of black and Asian clients to art therapy. I carried out an audit of referrals over two years and compared the numbers with the client base of the team. I found that my hunch was right, so I then engaged with the team to look at reasons why and how referrals might be increased. I also noticed that I was receiving fewer referrals of men than women, although the service as a whole worked with equal numbers of both genders. The defining standard here was the offer of art therapy equally to all groups being cared for by the team. There are of course many other aspects of work to audit, e.g. time taken to process referrals, client satisfaction, and so on.

Another example of a possible audit concerned uptake of a ten-session anger management art therapy group. I ran two groups, three years apart. Both groups started with roughly equal numbers of men and women, but each time most of the women dropped out, while most of the men stayed the course. Clearly the service met the men's needs but not the women's. If the groups had been closer together in time, a useful audit would have been to ask the women their reasons for dropping out. These may have been to do with the style of the group, the presence of men, domestic or other reasons. This would be useful information in planning future groups, with the aim of providing a service to meet both men's and women's needs in this area.

Evidence-based practice and quantitative research

Evidence-based healthcare is defined as the conscientious, explicit and judicious use of current best evidence in making decisions abut any aspects of healthcare (Li Wan Po 1998). Research is therefore designed to produce new findings and test new hypotheses, producing results that can be generalised. This seems like common sense. Everyone wants their clients to have treatments that are 'known to work'. In a climate of increasing financial pressure, there is a need for managers to make the best use of the funds available and therefore to favour 'proven' treatments. However, it is not that simple to prove what works, which can be defined in many ways, and research can be lengthy and expensive.

For any kind of research, considerable preparation is needed, such as a literature search, application to an ethics committee, research design and pilot, statistical methods advice, and so on. In the NHS all research must involve service users, from the design stage to implementation and follow-up. This section covers the two main quantitative methods of research: randomised controlled trials and outcome studies.

Randomised controlled trials

Randomised controlled trials (RCTs) are regarded in many fields as the 'gold standard' for scientific proof of clinical effectiveness. The purpose of this method is to remove any possible bias by carrying out any measures (e.g. a new therapy) on one group (randomly chosen from the total target group) and comparing the results with a control group. Goldner and Blisker (1995) outline the 'rules of evidence':

- an explicit hypothesis/research question
- reliable and valid measures
- random allocation of subjects
- statistical evaluation
- large samples
- blind experimenters and/or subjects
- measures are specific and sensitive to the variable being measured.

Evidence-based medicine was pioneered in Canada in the 1980s and its application to psychotherapy in the UK was highlighted by the NHS review of strategic policy on psychotherapy services in England (DoH 1996). This review recommended investing in services meeting the following five standards:

1   Clinical guidelines adopted for standard practice.
2   Guidelines informed by research and service evaluation.

3   Appropriate services specified for particular patient groups.
4   Outcomes for innovative treatments monitored.
5   Key elements of standard practice audited (Parry 2000: 59–60).

In practice, these strict scientific guidelines are difficult to apply to subjective data and to processes where meaning is often more important than objective 'symptoms'. Moreover the large sample needed makes such research difficult to achieve without considerable resources. Regarding art therapy, we have not yet found a way to take into account the complexity of the artwork produced. Many people are quite critical of evidence-based practice (EBP) in its narrow approach (Parry 2000), especially as scientific research itself rarely leads to clear unequivocal answers. There is also the point that 'no evidence' does not mean that something does not work, simply that the research has not been done. There are many commonly accepted practices (including medical ones) which have not been tested by an RCT. Despite the inherent difficulties, there have been a few attempts at RCTs involving art therapy. Here is a brief account of a recent research project:

> This study assessed the likely incremental benefit of art therapy over a standard package of community mental health team (CMHT) care when used with mental health service users with a diagnosis of schizophrenia. 90 mental health service users currently in active contact with community mental health teams were randomised to ongoing standard CMHT care – consisting of regular medication review and contact with a community psychiatric nurse – or CMHT care plus 12 weekly sessions of interactive group art therapy. Patients were assessed on a range of measures of symptoms, interpersonal interaction and psychosocial functioning at pre-treatment, post-treatment and three months follow up.
>
> The study found that there was significant improvement for clients receiving brief art therapy plus CMHT care on the Scale for the Assessment of Negative Symptoms (SANS; Andreasen 1989). This scale showed a statistically significant improvement at post therapy and six months follow up. There was a general trend toward positive outcome on the other measures.
>
> The RCT is often described as 'laboratory work' and counterpoised to the 'messy' realities of clinical experience. In the recruitment phase of this RCT, the clinician and research assistants went out into the community and visited people in their homes. This brought them into direct contact with the realities of deprivation, illness and inequality faced by many people with this diagnosis in a way which was not usual in routine clinical practice. The RCT also recruited approximately 27% more black and minority ethnic clients to the art therapy groups than was the case for art therapy groups provided by the art therapy service

of the NHS trust in which the RCT took place. This quantitative increase in numbers of black and minority ethnic clients reflected a qualitative improvement in access to art therapy services during the RCT for black and minority ethnic clients.

(Jones 2002)

Outcome studies

Some of these have already been referred to above, under Evaluation Involving Group Members, p. 58. There are also many other kinds of outcomes which can be researched in a quantitative way, such as hospital admission rates, self harm incidents, attendance rates at groups, and so on. There are many different research designs which can be adopted. Outcome studies can form the whole or part of a research design.

There are of course, many other research methods, such as systematic reviews, non-random trials, case control studies, cohort studies, to mention a few, but these are beyond the scope of this book.

Evidence-based practice and qualitative research

Research is the systematic study of data and observations, with a view to answering a particular question. As well as drawing on scientific methods (as in EBP), art therapists draw on psychological methods (e.g. outcome studies) and arts methods (e.g. case studies, historical research, picture reviews). All of these provide evidence of their own kind and a research design may include several different methods. Often quantitative research (such as RCTs and outcome studies) needs to be accompanied by qualitative studies to provide depth to the findings. Below is a list of some types of qualitative research commonly used to evaluate the effects of art therapy. Some of these can be used to obtain both quantitative and qualitative data.

Case studies

This is the most commonly used form of research as it most closely follows therapeutic practice. In groupwork, it is possible to follow a group member through a series of sessions; or to study the development of the whole group; or to focus on emerging themes in the group. Even single-case research designs can be used to provide evidence (McNiff 1998: 159–67).

Personal documents

These can be collected in many different ways: diaries, written accounts, pictures and other artworks, photographs, videos, poems, narratives, biographies, and so on. They can all contribute evidence in their own way.

Written questionnaires

These are easy to use but sometimes difficult to get returned. They need to be clear, jargon free and fairly short, to encourage completion. Questions should follow through in a logical order (Ingram 2002a). A letter outlining the purpose and a stamped addressed envelope help. They are useful in situations where interviews are not feasible or appropriate, e.g. follow-up responses to a group, or finding information on similar groups in other parts of the country.

Interviews

These are usually carried out by an independent person using a semi-structured or open-ended questionnaire, which gives a focus to the discussion but leaves enough room for people to give their views, especially if there is a 'catch-all' question at the end. Questionnaires should be piloted to make sure they are clear and give the information you are looking for. Such interviews often give a wealth of information not achievable by written questionnaires on their own. It is good to tape them, but remember they take time to transcribe (about seven hours for one hour of interview). Telephone interviews can also be used but result in much less information. Service users can often be good interviewers as they may be able to build up better rapport with interviewees.

Focus groups

These are small groups of people (six to eight) who come together to give their views. Discussion may help to clarify opinions and issues. Many of the considerations of interviews apply here. In addition, group management skills are needed (Ingram 2002b).

Action research

This kind of research acknowledges the effect of the researcher's actions on the research and includes it in the research design (Payne 1993). It can be used to encourage change within a particular setting (McNiff 1998).

Collaborative or partnership research

This type of research is influenced by the subjects' and the researcher's values, motivations and methods. It is designed and developed in collaboration with the research subjects (Payne 1993).

Art-based research

This is not a totally separate category from all the others, but a reminder that art therapy is based on visual processes, which can therefore provide an appropriate basis for research (McNiff 1998). McNiff points out that the process of art often uncovers something different from the reasoning mind (p.77), so it has the potential to provide another route to research. He provides 76 examples of possible research and evaluation designs based on art processes, in different categories (effects of aesthetic quality, method studies, histories, outcome assessments).

This is also where visual methods of recording have a place, such as photography and video (as mentioned in the section on Recording, pp. 53–6). The use of digital cameras makes it possible to analyse almost frame by frame the visual development of artwork, as in a recent article by Richard Lanham (2002).

Whatever the research design, all research needs to conform to regulatory issues in research governance, such as rigour, review, data protection, monitoring and publication. For more details, see *Information for Research Governance* (DoH 2001).

Practice research networks

The emphasis on evidence-based practice and research has led to the formation of practice research networks (PRNs), which are networks of clinicians who agree to collaborate to collect data through routine clinical practice rather than special research trials. They try to use the same measures and data collection tools, so that they can collect large sets of data and make comparisons (Barkham and Mellor-Clark 2000).

An Art Therapy Practice Research Network (ATPRN) was set up by Val Huet and Neil Springham in 2000 to initiate the building of networks among art therapists who want to undertake and learn about practice-based evaluation and research. It explores research strategies for art therapy, disseminates ideas and skills, and provides support for art therapists who are both practitioners and researchers. The network meets twice yearly in London and once yearly in Scotland. It has special interest groups that focus on clinical specialisms, e.g. older adults, children and adolescents, psychosis, trauma. Recent projects have included ideas about collaborative research projects and a 'banding' project to audit the level of severity of clients seen by art therapists nationally. A website is planned to help practitioners to connect with others researching their area of practice. The address is in the Resources section (ATPRN 2002a, 2002b).

Art therapy research register

This has been prepared to appear in Gilroy (2003) and includes a list of all art therapy research to date in the UK, both completed and ongoing. The list will also be made available separately through BAAT (AT Newsbriefing 2002).

Conclusion

This chapter has given an overview of methods of recording, evaluation and research. It is not meant to be a daunting menu required of therapists and facilitators, rather a list of possibilities with signposts to further resources, as the need and opportunity arises. These can be found in the References below and in the Resources section at the end of the book.

References

Andreasen, N. (1989) 'Scale for the assessment of negative symptoms', *British Journal of Psychiatry*, 155, 7: 49–53.

AT Newsbriefing (2002) 'Art therapy research register', June: 12.

ATPRN (2002a) 'ATPRN report to the 2002 BAAT AGM', *AT Newsbriefing*, September: 1.

ATPRN (2002b) Notice, *AT Newsbriefing*, December: 1.

Barkham, M. and Mellor-Clark, J. (2000) 'Rigour and relevance: the role of practice-based evidence in the psychological therapies', in N. Rowland and S. Goss (eds) *Evidence-Based Counselling and Psychological Therapies: Research and Applications*, London: Routledge.

Case, C. and Dalley, T. (1992) *The Handbook of Art Therapy*, London: Tavistock/ Routledge.

Clinical Effectiveness Support Unit (CESU) (1997) *Clinical Effectiveness and the Therapy Professions: Resource File*, Cardiff: CESU.

Corcos, N. (2002) 'Solutions in art therapy: toward a visual outcome measure', paper delivered at Theoretical Advances of Art Therapy Conference, 19 October, University of Aston, Birmingham. Abstract on website: <www.baat.org/taoat/ corcos_2002.html> (further details from Nadija Corcos, Long Fox Unit, Weston General Hospital, Grange Road, Weston-super-Mare, Somerset BS23 4TQ).

Cox, M. (1988) *Coding the Therapeutic Process*, London: Jessica Kingsley Publishers.

Department of Health (DoH) (1996) *A Review of Strategic Policy on NHS Psychotherapy Services in England* (ed. G. Parry), London: NHS Executive.

Department of Health (DoH) (2001) *Information for Research Governance*, London: DoH. Website: <www.researchinformation.nhs.uk/main/governance.htm>

Gantt, L. and Tabone, C. (1998) *Formal Elements Art Therapy Scale Manual*, West Virginia: Gargoyle Press.

George, E., Iveson, I. and Ratner, H. (1999) *Problem to Solution: Brief Therapy with Individuals and Families*, London: BT Press.

Gilroy, A. (2003) *Art Therapy, Research and Evidence Based Practice*, London: Sage.

Goldner, E. M. and Bliskor, D. (1995) 'Evidence-based practice in psychiatry', *Canadian Journal of Psychiatry*, 40, 2: 97–101.

Healy, K. (1998) 'Clinical audit and conflict', in R. Davenhill and M. Patrick (eds) *Rethinking Clinical Audit: The Case of Psychotherapy Services in the NHS*, London: Routledge.

Ingram, J. (2002a) 'Questionnaire design', lecture notes, Research & Development Support Unit (RSDU), United Bristol Healthcare Trust.

Ingram, J. (2002b) 'Introduction to qualitative methods', lecture notes, Research & Development Support Unit (RSDU), United Bristol Healthcare Trust.

Jones, K. (2002) 'A randomised controlled trial (RCT) of group based brief art therapy', paper delivered at Theoretical Advances of Art Therapy Conference, 19 October. Abstract on website: <www.baat.org/taoat/jones_2002.html> (further details from Kevin Jones, Art Psychotherapy course, Goldsmith's College, 23 St James, London SE14 6NW).

Lanham, R. (2002) 'Inscape revisited', *Inscape*, Seven, 2: 48–59.

Lewis, S. and Williams, F. (2002) 'Witnesses to the unutterable: developing an assessment tool for use in art therapy practice', work in progress.

Li Wan Po, A. (1998) *Dictionary of Evidence Based Medicine*, Abingdon: Radcliffe Medical Press.

McDowell, I. and Newell, C. (1996) *Measuring Health: Guide to Rating Scales and Questionnaires*, 2nd edn, Oxford: Oxford University Press.

McNiff, S. (1998) *Art-Based Research*, London: Jessica Kingsley Publishers.

Manners, R. (1998) *The Arts Therapies Service: Clinical Protocol (Pilot – May 1998)*, Cwmbran: Gwent Community Health NHS Trust.

National Health Service (NHS) (1999a) *National Service Framework for Mental Health*, London: Department of Health. Website: <www.doh.gov.uk/nsf/mentalhealth.htm>

National Health Service (NHS) (1999b) *Clinical Governance: Quality in the New NHS*, London: NHS Executive. Website: <www.doh.gov.uk/clinicalgovernance>

Ogles, B. M., Lambert, M. J. and Field, S. A. (2002) *Essentials of Outcome Measurement*, New York: Wiley.

Parry, G. (1996) 'Service evaluation and audit methods', in G. Parry and F. N. Watts (eds) *Behavioural and Mental Health Research: A Handbook of Skills and Methods*, Hove: Lawrence Erlbaum Associates Ltd.

Parry, G. (2000) 'Evidence-based psychotherapy: an overview' in N. Rowland and S. Goss (eds) *Evidence-Based Counselling and Psychological Therapies: Research and Applications*, London: Routledge.

Payne, H. (1993) 'From practitioner to researcher: research as a learning process', in H. Payne (ed.) *Handbook of Inquiry in the Arts Therapies: One River, Many Currents*, London: Jessica Kingsley Publishers.

Sharry, J. (2001) *Solution-Focused Groupwork*, London: Sage.

South West MIND (1996) *Avon Mental Health Measure: A User-Centred Approach to Assessing Need*, Bristol: MIND.

Whitaker, D. S. (2001) *Using Groups to Help People*, 2nd edn, London: Brunner-Routledge.

Wood, C. (1999) 'Gathering evidence: expansion of art therapy research strategy', *Inscape*, Four, 2: 51–61.

Chapter 4

Learning from problems in groups

Personal art and art therapy groups that take place in real life are much messier than the ideal versions laid out in theory. Although there are aspects that can be predicted (for instance, that most people will be anxious about the first group meeting), there is always an element of unpredictability because no one is ever in full possession of all the relevant facts, and therapists and facilitators are not infinitely wise. Even if one could satisfy these impossible conditions, there are always outside factors that could not have been foreseen. However, even some of the imperfections can be turned to good advantage, and the resulting groups can be very satisfying experiences which add significantly to individuals' growth and development. The most important thing is to be able to learn from problem situations and mistakes.

One way of approaching this subject would be to go through all the aspects of running a group mentioned in Chapter 2 and imagine the effect on the group of the lack of each requirement; e.g. difficult physical arrangements, interruptions, lack of support from other staff, inappropriate referrals, disruptive individuals, inexperienced leaders, bad introductions, poorly chosen themes, and so on. Rather than spell out the consequences of these, I would like to give some examples of difficulties experienced by art therapists in a variety of groups. They are taken from interviews with several art therapists, mostly with considerable experience and working in a wide variety of settings, talking honestly about groups they have facilitated. I have grouped the quotations under five headings which reflect commonly experienced problems. It is important to note that these problems are described from the therapists' and facilitators' points of view. Under each heading I quote the examples first and then comment on them. Some of these comments apply specifically to one example, others apply to several of the examples.

Outside factors

Example 1

'On one ward, I arrived to find they were redecorating the usual room we use. The only place we could go was the dining-room next door; we tried to hold the group there, but other people kept wandering through. It was terrible. We never really got started, and in the end we just packed up.'

Example 2

'Initially staff on the long-stay ward were suspicious of art therapy sessions, seemed not to want their patients to be "over-stimulated"! There was no co-operation and they resisted allowing the patients to attend. However, on seeing the products of the sessions, staff attitudes have changed and they are now keen for them to come.'

Comments

Example 1 describes just one of many unsuitable venues in which therapists and facilitators may find themselves working. It is sometimes difficult to decide whether it is worth carrying on, or whether the environment is so unsuitable that it is best to call a halt. Guiding factors will be whether the group is providing more benefits than problems to clients and members, and whether there is some hope that conditions can be improved in the future. Often there is more leverage at the start of a programme or group, when staff and managers may be more ready to listen to what is needed, so it is worth being clear about the needs of the group and asking for the facilities. The lists in Chapter 2, Setting up the group, should help with this.

Example 2 shows the importance of getting staff on board. This can be done in several ways. One way is to run a workshop for staff before setting out with clients, so that there is some awareness of the process and the benefits. If this is too exposing for staff, giving a talk and showing pictures or slides of other clients' work (with their permission) can demonstrate what the work is about. Finally, seeing the effects of the work in their setting often convinces staff of the value of this work. One way of gaining allies is to invite other staff to co-facilitate groups. For instance, in a community mental health team, I have seen several community psychiatric nurses completely revise their opinion of art therapy after such an experience.

Co-facilitator problems

Example 3

'Sometimes when staff [in a day centre for older people] participate in the group, they take over and start telling people what to do, so I mostly prefer to run the group on my own.'

Example 4

'A visiting art therapist got into a confrontation with a group member. It wasn't resolved and was all left in the air. Later I realised it was up to me, as co-facilitator, to stop the group and point out that a misunderstanding had arisen over the use of a word which has come to have a special meaning at our centre, which the visiting therapist couldn't have known. I suppose we should have sorted out our roles beforehand; while the visiting art therapist was in charge of the process, I, as co-facilitator, could have been ready to clarify any confusions.'

Comments

Example 3 demonstrates the frustration that can occur in using untrained staff as co-facilitators. In some institutions this can happen because of shortage of staff and lack of understanding about art therapy. In a day centre for older people, there is probably little risk attached to sole working as there will be other staff nearby, and older people are not as likely as some other client groups to behave in a volatile way. But for many groups the solution of sole working would be an unsafe one, either because of the building or because of the client group. I myself had to postpone a group (in a community mental health team) when my co-facilitator got another job and there was no one to take his place for some months. In a ten-week group with volatile members, another facilitator was needed to cope with sudden outbursts and people leaving the group. For this particular group we also needed a male and a female facilitator/therapist.

The lessons of Example 4 are all too clear. It is essential for co-therapists to prepare well beforehand together and to clarify their roles. It is not always easy to stop the group in the middle, depending on the client group and their needs. If the group is meeting over several sessions, another way of dealing with this is to wait until the end of the session and then clarify roles and assumptions with each other. As well as preparing specifically for the session, it is also vital to share assumptions about therapy, as direct confrontations with group members can be destructive unless handled very sensitively. It can be more constructive to open up such issues to the whole group.

Disruptive group members

Example 5

'In one of my groups of elderly people, there was a woman who could not stop talking and other people couldn't concentrate on what they were doing. I tried to control it, but that only made it worse. There always seem to be one or two like that in my groups, and it makes me feel very tense, which in turn makes things worse. I don't like excluding people for that reason because that's what they need help in.'

Example 6

'If someone is known to be disruptive, I don't include them. I used to, but not any more. I also exclude people if past experience shows they will not get anything out of the art therapy groups.'

Example 7

'When Graham arrived an hour late, everyone was at their peak of concentration. He seemed quite unaware of the effect of his entry, and started to talk immediately, so I hustled him into the kitchen for a cup of tea, and to bring him up to date with what we were doing. I asked him not to talk while painting, and not to be late next week.' (Community group meeting in a church hall, see Chapter 5.)

Example 8

'I find it's difficult sometimes to handle one person's particular problem in the group, if it's not shared by others – for instance, grief.'

Comments

These examples describe the dilemmas and some of the solutions chosen to deal with disruptive group members – those people whose contributions seem to impede the group's functioning. Of course the label disruptive may be a matter of opinion, and each group and therapist may have different ideas about what is regarded as disruptive. Examples 5 and 7 show an understanding that the very fact of being disruptive is one reason why people need the group, so that therapists are reluctant to exclude people. Often therapists and facilitators do not have the luxury of knowing in advance if someone is going to be disruptive. It becomes all too apparent only when the group has started. A way of deciding whether to include known disruptive people or not is whether their presence is going to be so disruptive that no one else can gain any benefit. I have occasionally spotted this at pre-group interviews and asked people to observe certain conditions, such as trying to speak about the problem rather than victimising someone else in the group. Even so, I have sometimes wondered if the group might have been better for others if I had excluded certain people at the beginning. Sometimes a good way forward is to involve the rest of the group in discussing how the behaviour affects them and how the group can proceed. It can be difficult to decide when this is the best course, when it is better to accept the behaviour, and when someone needs to be excluded.

Example 8 is not so much about a disruptive group member but about a situation in which there is a member who has a problem not shared by others. Although this is difficult, it may be possible to build bridges with other members by focusing on the things they do have are in common; for instance, that from time to time we all have problems that make us feel we are on our own – or in the case of grief, we have all suffered some kind of loss. Even groups set up to deal with particular problems or to include similar clients will be comprised of a wide variety of people who may or may not have a lot in common. Often other group members will be sympathetic to a person with a different problem and give them the time they need. It can be an opportunity for group members to empathise with others and offer help.

Strong feelings evoked in the group

Example 9

'I used to think my groups had gone wrong if anyone burst into tears and left the room. Now I provide a big box of tissues and accept tears as part of the group as they are part of life. If someone wants to leave the room for a bit, or rushes out, my co-facilitator sits with them until they are ready to come back in or decide to go home.'

Example 10

'Strong feelings can be evoked by some themes; for instance, feelings of conflict, confrontation, loss, hurt, rejection. But if people are experiencing these feelings anyway, I feel it's better to find a way of dealing with them than just to miss them all out, though I would hope to approach them gradually.'

Example 11

'Group paintings are not always predictable; they can sometimes highlight the difficulties between people. But sharing these can help towards resolution.'

Example 12

'I was quite upset by the amount of aggression and hostility that came out in the group painting done by the women's group, in particular between two individuals. Previously I'd had the illusion everyone got on with each other. Later I learned that the two women in particular conflict had met for lunch the next week to talk about their differences, so the group had in fact been beneficial.'

Example 13

'Messy feelings are better than an artificial calm which may be rigid and superficial.'

Example 14

'If all the group members are depressed and turned in on themselves, the group can feel very flat and I seem to get little back. But I think I may underestimate what happens, as sometimes I find out later people have still got something out of it.'

Comments

All these examples describe moments in personal art or art therapy groups where strong feelings arise. Doing the artwork does often make it more likely that these feelings arise, but it also provides a vehicle to help deal with them too. When strong feelings are evoked, there is the opportunity to explore them and work towards some kind of resolution. The pictures can also act as containers for the feelings, and the act of putting them away at the end of a session can be a metaphor for handling the feelings. They can be expressed, explored and then left in a safe place until the next session.

Learning from experience

Example 15

'A lot went wrong in my first year because I was nervous and tense. I was trying to control the group, and appointed myself as its protector.'

Example 16

'Certain themes can be threatening for certain groups, and I have tried to learn to be sensitive to the individuals in the groups, and introduce themes which can be developed on different levels. I have learnt that preparation time is really important.'

Example 17

'It's very easy to miss quite important messages. After a group which had painted early childhood memories, one woman asked me what could go wrong if children had no mother. I answered this at face value and quoted research about maternal deprivation. Later I realised that, as she was a cancer patient, she was probably expressing in an indirect way her worry about dying and leaving her children bereft. I could have kicked myself for the extra burden I had given her. If I had been more perceptive I could have allayed her fears by referring to further research on mother-substitutes. I am now rather wiser about the way people often ask their most important questions indirectly, because it is too threatening to do so directly.'

Example 18

'Two days after learning about the conversation above, someone in a community group asked me how art therapy helped mental patients. Before launching into a great thesis on the topic, I enquired a bit further about what she really wanted to know. It turned out that she had been in hospital herself, and had been worried about her lack of ability to paint there. I and others tried to reassure her about this. I was very grateful to have been able to learn from someone else's mistake, so that I could avoid further hurting someone.'

Example 19

'One of the members of my group did a painting which included me. He was very angry with me, and I realised that I was part of his world at that moment. He was seeing me in a parental role. I had to acknowledge that before we could go on.'

Example 20

'I got into an argument with a group member over his picture of a brick wall. I think he was setting me up. Perhaps if I had used more imagination we might have avoided the impasse.'

Comments

Even experienced therapists and facilitators make mistakes, as the quotations in this section demonstrate. This is not the end of the world, providing one can learn from one's mistakes and times of insensitivity. All these examples show some learning that has taken place as the result of experience.

In Examples 15, 17 and 20 there is a realisation of how previous ways of reacting had been counterproductive, and Examples 16 and 19 show how learning has resulted in new ways of handling group tasks. Example 19 shows an awareness of transference issues. Example 18 shows how it is possible to transfer learning from one situation to another, and from one person to another. One does not have to make all the mistakes oneself in order to progress.

When to intervene in a group

It is often difficult to decide when to intervene in a group and when not to. It is a good idea to intervene if:

- it opens up opportunities for effective work
- something needs dealing with
- damage is being done to an individual.

It is best not to intervene if:

- members are doing good work themselves
- the intervention won't be heard
- you are not clear what is happening yet (Whitaker 2001: 238–40).

Conclusion

As can be seen from some of the examples given, it is not always obvious whether a difficult session was a group where things went wrong or the beginning of growth and development for that group or individuals in it. A little time needs to be allowed before coming to any such conclusion, and indeed the therapist or facilitator may never know the outcome.

It is worth investing in one or two books on groupwork, so that when problems arise (as they inevitably do) you can reflect on a variety of ways forward, and choose the most appropriate for your group and situation. There are several good groupwork books which outline problem situations in a systematic way in much greater detail than is possible here. *Using Groups to Help People* (Whitaker 2001) has a chapter devoted to problems and opportunities, including many examples, with thoughtful commentaries on possible courses of action. *Groupwork* (Brown 1992) lists a range of options for responding to individual behaviour, with some special techniques to counteract scapegoating.

There are many ways of reflecting on one's own practice: by sharing difficult experiences with colleagues and people doing similar work in other places; by obtaining good and regular supervision, preferably from an experienced group art therapist; by attending appropriate training courses.

In an imperfect world, there is certainly room for the idea of the 'good enough' facilitator or therapist, who does his or her best to avoid pitfalls, can learn from them when they occur, and in general has a thoughtful, positive and caring approach to the group and its members.

References

Brown, A. (1992) *Groupwork*, 3rd edn, Aldershot: Ashgate.

Whitaker, D. S. (2001) *Using Groups to Help People*, 2nd edn, London: Brunner-Routledge.

Chapter 5

An example in detail

The 'Friday Group'

I have chosen this particular example for several reasons. First, it is one that I was directly involved in and for which I kept notes at the time, so the details and atmosphere remain fresh. It was an ongoing group so it shows the group process over a period of time and how the nature of a group can change. It was a group that took place in the community, so was not bound to any one kind of therapeutic situation (and also had some difficulties arising from that fact). Finally, one or two of the sessions (which I shall describe in detail) demonstrate how widely certain themes can be interpreted by individuals. The group was started by a friend of mine, Heather (a trained art therapist), to explore two of her particular interests to see if they could be related:

(a) colour work;
(b) the psychology of personal construct theory (Burr and Butt 1992; Dalton and Dunnett 1999; Fransella 1995), as developed by George Kelly (1963).

The group was called an 'Art and Psychology Study-Workshop' and was advertised by notices in relevant magazines and posters in suitable places.

The group met on Friday mornings from 10.00 am–1.30 pm in a hired church room, with a kitchen next door where we could make drinks. I was to be part of the group as I was not familiar with Heather's chosen topics and also to act as co-facilitator when required. At the beginning I interpreted this as helping the people who came together to feel at home and welcome.

A mixed group of people arrived for the first session. Some had come as a substitute for another workshop which had fallen through, some via posters and advertisements, some via personal contacts. The initial group included a couple practising alternative therapies, two semi-retired women, three women with young children (two of whom had previously taught art and crafts), myself and Heather. Over the next few weeks, during the initial phase, the couple and one of the older women left and we were joined for varying numbers of sessions by a retired doctor, a playgroup leader, two unemployed men, an osteopath, a woman with older children and an unemployed art therapist new to the city. The attendance varied from two to eight, depending on such things as sick children, visits of relatives and the weather (it often rained torrentially on Fridays, we noticed, as we struggled in and out of the building with paints, paper, jars, etc.).

Because we were meeting in a church room that was used by many other groups, Heather had to bring all the materials every week in her estate car, which she unloaded while parked momentarily on the double yellow lines of the busy main road outside. She had to bring everything: paints, paper, brushes, palettes, water jars, newsprint rolls to cover the tables, newspaper to spread on the floor for paintings to dry, rags, paper tissues, books which might be of interest to the group. Heather also had to organise the room each week: take up the carpet in the middle of the floor, bring in some small formica-topped tables from the lobby and put them together to make a large painting surface, put out all the materials (Figure 5.1 shows the group at work). Although Heather usually got there early to set everything out, members of the group naturally helped to clear away at the end.

The first eight sessions had a similar format. We started with a cup of tea and any introductions. Then Heather introduced a colour exercise, loosely based on some of Rudolf Steiner's work, using wet paper and water colours in particular sequences. (For an introduction to Steiner's Anthroposophical

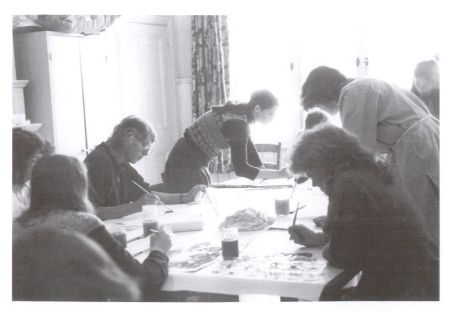

Figure 5.1   The 'Friday Group' at work (Bristol Art and Psychology Group)
Source: Photograph by Marian Liebmann

approaches, see Part II, Section J, no. 351.) We discussed the results and
then had a short break for lunch, after which Heather introduced some of
Kelly's personal construct theories. The atmosphere was much like that of
an informal adult education class, but more personal because the subject
matter was personal and the group was fairly small.

When the group had settled down, people began to talk to each other
more and to ask more questions. Knowing we were both art therapists,
people asked us about this too, so Heather asked the group if they would
like to try some 'art therapy' themes, which they did.

Earliest childhood memory

This was taken together with the first memory of separation and hellos and
goodbyes in the present to see if there were any connections between past
and present. The results were interesting. Jenny did a picture of herself and
her sister being sent off to nursery school. Most of the picture was in black
to emphasise the misery of separation.

Audrey painted the occasion when she dawdled on a walk and the others
went on without her. She knelt down, bellowed with rage and wailed, 'Wait
for me!' Her parents must have thought it was funny as her father took a
photograph of her, but she was actually very angry and frightened.

My painting showed me visiting my mother in hospital when my younger
brother was born, but somehow I couldn't seem to remember much – a lot
seemed to be 'blotted out'.

We all found the theme unexpectedly upsetting, as if a lot of our childhood hurts were still all there, if we 'pressed the right buttons'. It certainly
convinced us that we had not entirely forgotten our early experiences.
Although the present-day experiences did not always dovetail into these, we
began to see that there might be strands of earlier experiences still influ-
encing us.

Family groups in clay

Heather asked us to model a family group. It was the only time we used
clay (mainly because of the practicalities of bringing it and of taking home
any finished articles). One or two people found it difficult initially. Everyone worked away with deep concentration. Then we shared our thoughts
and feelings.

Audrey

A family group including herself, her husband and two baby girls, with her
mother nearby.

Ruth

Three figures rising from a unified base, arms flowing between each member as if dancing or rotating, the balance of the group disturbed by the removal of the fourth member. (Ruth's marriage had recently broken up, and her husband had moved out, leaving her looking after their two young children.)

Tamsin

Four figures on the same base, representing an 'idealised family' she had never known in her childhood.

Jenny

A large number of small figures, lots of brothers and sisters, everyone's children, all coming and going.

Myself

My own small family in the centre, surrounded by a circle of friends, who for us take the place of the large family we haven't got.

Most of us thoroughly enjoyed using clay, except for Tamsin who felt it was cold and clammy. We found it interesting to see that there were many interpretations of 'family' other than our own and how using clay enabled us to express these in a way that neither words nor pictures could manage.

The group membership

A couple of sessions later Heather was away so I took responsibility for the group for that session. By now the membership had settled down.

Audrey

She was a retired teacher doing voluntary work at the local cancer help centre and very interested in using art in a personal way. She and her husband seemed to have some difficulties.

Jenny

A mother of two young children, she had also done quite a lot of sessional craft teaching. Her husband had been unemployed for a long time and was very depressed on account of this. The family was living on social security and Jenny naturally found their situation difficult and depressing.

Ruth

A mother of two young children and former art teacher in a secondary school, in her teaching she had been searching for a more personal approach. Her marriage had recently broken up leaving her on her own with the children, living on benefits and having arguments with her ex-husband over financial arrangements. She felt very angry about him and this often spilled over into other interactions.

Lesley

She was a friend of Ruth's, in her second marriage and mother of one child. She was unable to continue coming when she got a part-time job.

Mary

A playgroup leader with grown-up children, she was unable to continue coming when her mother-in-law became ill and she had to look after her.

Myself

A mother of one child, an art therapist and working part time in another job I was trying to leave and looking for the right next step.

Heather

An art therapist working part time in several different places: a day hospital, a cancer help centre and a school for learning disabled children.

Then we were joined by two new members who rapidly became part of the group:

Pippa

A friend of Audrey's and a mother of three school-age children, her main love was painting, which she did in a very lively and vivid way.

Graham

A middle-aged man whose marriage had split up and whose son was at boarding school. He had been unemployed for a long time, and was trying to set up on his own, running a magazine about his main interest – astrology. He was a very lonely person and couldn't stop talking, while at the same time finding it difficult to make personal contact with others.

Because of the newcomers, I wanted to suggest a theme that would help me (and the rest of the group) get to know them, and at the same time be interesting and useful to those who knew each other. So after our usual initial cup of tea and exchange of greetings we sat down round the table and, as we were an 'established' group, I introduced the idea fairly directly, together with one or two other themes, so that the group had a choice and felt they had some say in what we did.

Lifelines

I asked people to draw or paint their life as a line and include, if they wished, any scenes or particular moments along the way. The line could be any shape. They could use large or small paper and sellotape extra sheets on if they needed. We had powder colours (Heather was using the liquid paints elsewhere that day), oil pastels and wax crayons at our disposal.

With eight of us in the room, space was at a premium. There was room for four people comfortably round the main table and two of us got some children's tables out at each end of the room. Ruth sellotaped her paper to the door of a metal cupboard and Jenny moved from the table to the floor when the number of sheets she needed outgrew her space on the table.

Everyone worked with great concentration for an hour, interrupted by Graham who arrived in the middle in a great flurry. I gave him a cup of tea in the kitchen and told him what we were doing. I decided to join in as everyone seemed to be engrossed and not to need anything. My style generally is to join in unless there are other things that need doing. As people worked, they spread on to more and more sheets of paper. When I saw that some had finished while others were still engrossed, I suggested that we had an early lunch break and met again in half an hour. This would give those still working the option of using some of that time to carry on if they wished.

After the break we gathered again. As the paintings were all different shapes and sizes, we moved round the room as a group to visit each painting. They were all fascinatingly different and for this reason I have included photographs of them (not all to the same scale). I asked who would like to start and no one volunteered, so I asked Graham, who was usually very talkative. After that, we just followed round the pictures in the order of the room.

Graham

As Graham had arrived late, he hadn't finished. His lifeline (no photograph available) was in the shape of a circle, as he believed in reincarnation. Within the circle he had placed some colours, a house, logs, a lake, which he thought of as 'life resources', and then a grey and brown cell representing his present home life, which he felt was pretty barren since splitting up from his wife. His son was at boarding school. He wanted to take it home and finish it.

Pippa

Pippa's lifeline (Figure 5.2) was a meandering blue river which wandered through exotic landscapes, replete with luscious fruits and brightly coloured flowers. Her parents had been diplomats and had taken her to several Middle Eastern countries, and there had been holidays with Danish grandparents too. The little vignettes along the way showed the Danish forests, a ripe juicy persimmon held in two hands, a little Middle Eastern playmate with black teeth, herself praying in a secret shrine she had made in a cave and her passion for riding. Although she had stuck two pieces of paper together, her lifeline only took her as far as the age of 11. The richness of her picture suggested a particular attachment to that period and she said herself that in many ways she still felt like a child.

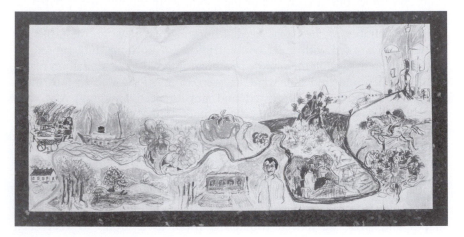

Figure 5.2   Lifeline: Pippa
Source: Photograph by David Newton

Mary

Mary (Figure 5.3) had sellotaped three sheets together. The first three represented her childhood, with rhythmic and uncomplicated wavy lines. The fourth piece was full of energetic whirls and brightly coloured shapes, with knots of darker colours here and there. These were to do with her eldest boy's hearing problems, and the arguments and difficulties with in-laws over her adoption of a child of part-Jamaican/part-Irish background.

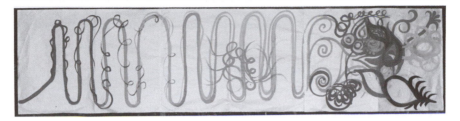

Figure 5.3   Lifeline: Mary
Source: Photograph by David Newton

Lesley

Lesley (Figure 5.4) had done an ingenious set of paintings in layers to represent her life. The bottom layer was painted in deep blue and purple to signify 'underlying' depression (lower picture, bottom right and left). On top of this, folded in towards the middle (bottom centre), was a layer depicting her childhood (the untidy dark mops), her teenage years (the cage) during which she had experienced a breakdown, and a white cross relating to her involvement with Christianity. The top layer (top picture), which was placed over the other two and also folded inwards, showed a huge white cross surrounded at the top by red and yellow, which she said were good things beginning to happen out of the nothingness below. She had done it in that way because she felt the top layers blotted out the memories of the others – were they gone, or just blotted out, she wondered? Right at the end, she did an oil pastel drawing showing a series of houses, each one progressively smaller. Her parents had moved around a lot, which she had found exciting at first. As more moves took place, the excitement palled and so she had drawn each house smaller. After the houses came a 'downward spiral' towards the bottom of the drawing, representing her difficult teenage years again.

Audrey

Audrey (Figure 5.5) started by drawing her lifeline (on two pieces of paper) as a large light-green spiral, which she said she would really have liked to do three-dimensionally, pointing upwards. The various scenes were significant events in her life, which she had jotted down in the top right-hand corner. The spiral started at the bottom left with her parents and her older brother at Audrey's birth. Higher up on the left is the birth of her much younger brother, whom she adored and virtually shared with her mother. Later followed her father's death from TB (bottom centre), depicted by a black hearse ('Free' was the name of the undertaker) and a sad circle of tearful heads. Further on (to right) were college days during the war

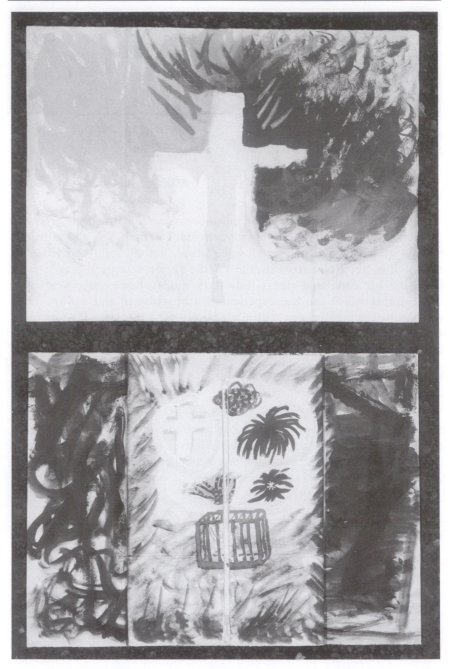

Figure 5.4   Lifeline: Lesley
Source: Photograph by David Newton

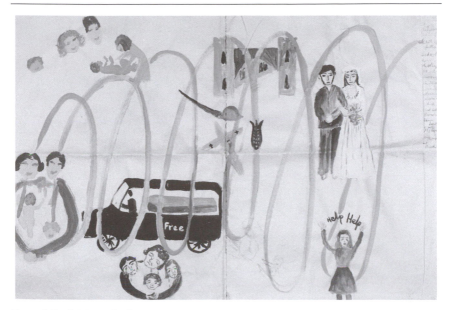

Figure 5.5 Lifeline: Audrey
Source: Photograph by David Newton

(castellated towers with sword, gun and helmet), followed by her wedding. The couple have quizzical expressions on their faces, she said, to signify the difficulties that were to come. In the bottom right she drew herself in her first job as a teacher, both with her pupils and on her own, shouting 'Help, Help!' because it was all too much for her at the time. As can be seen, she had not finished, so took it home to work on, in her deliberate and self-paced way. She also started a third piece of paper, but remarked that she felt the rest of her life was mostly not very eventful. As she was older than most of us, she felt that family life, once started, tended to go on for a long time much the same, and turning points would be difficult to find.

Ruth

Ruth did her picture in oil pastels (Figure 5.6), on two pieces of paper stuck to a metal cupboard door. Her art training is evident in her firm and organised use of materials. The colours she used were mostly pastel colours with some strong black lines and shapes. Starting at the top right, the large black question-mark remembered an occasion when, as a small child, she was abducted by a man. This was followed by an expanding bulbous portion, which showed her emerging from childhood. The square shape she related to a need for security, and the grey clouds inside to a period of

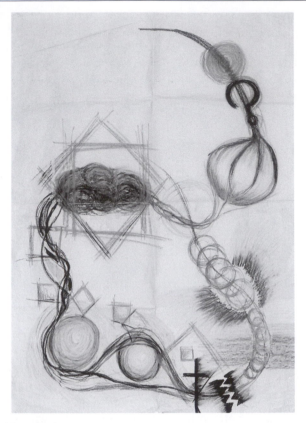

Figure 5.6   Lifeline: Ruth
Source: Photograph by David Newton

confusion at college. Black and brightly coloured lines worked their way towards the bottom of the picture, representing an 'unsubtle' marriage, and the two circles, pink and blue, stood for her children. At the lowest point a black cross was followed by a black jagged rift. The cross was for the sudden death of her sister, and the jagged rift for the break-up of her marriage. Both had happened quite recently, the latter only during the previous months. The smallish circles following on from this showed her working through the aftermath and leading upwards towards red and white wings for the present, where she felt she was 'taking off' again, in the direction of the top left of the picture.

Jenny

Jenny ended up using eight sheets of paper, spread out on the floor, as one thing led to another (Figure 5.7). Starting at the top left, with her birth (a spiral sun), the line shows her family as an inturned circle. They stayed in the same place all the time, whereas she would have liked to move around. She shocked them all by getting pregnant and having her son (small spiral sun) at the age of 17. She thoroughly enjoyed this, and it also helped her to make a lot of new contacts (little people at the top). She then met her husband (top right) and moved to various places with him (waves for a seaside resort, top right), including inner London, where they lived in communal housing with a central courtyard (bottom right) – the best place she'd ever lived. There followed a move to France (bottom centre), where they bought a derelict farmhouse with others and lived a basic, self-sufficient life in hard but rewarding conditions, and where her daughter was born. Then the line led back to Bristol (centre), a time of problems and complications, during which her youngest son was born, and finally finished on the left at the house they bought to 'settle down'. The bottom left flower shape was to represent the future, when she hoped to try to make interesting things happen from their base, without always having to move on.

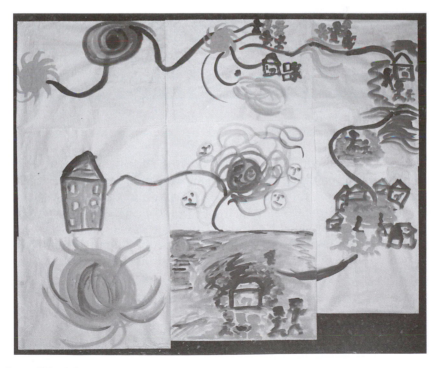

Figure 5.7 Lifeline: Jenny
Source: Photograph by David Newton

Myself

My lifeline spread on to four sheets of paper (Figure 5.8). Starting on the left, the first event depicted is the death of my father (prone figure), followed by a black line for difficult college days. This was followed by the discovery of painting and writing and a move to London (Underground sign), and then Bristol (coloured lights, a time of many contacts). Then another line joined mine, followed by a red blob (marriage) and a flowering of talents in a new job. The pear-shaped figure showed my pregnancy, and a third line joined us – a yellow one in between the two darker ones which twirled around as our young child led us a 'merry dance'. Below this was a black patch of depression associated with work and decision making, with arrows pointing in different directions I could take out of it. The little figure at the bottom was me looking over my shoulder, harking back to my favourite job. At the right was a green meadow, with flowers – a wish for an easier future.

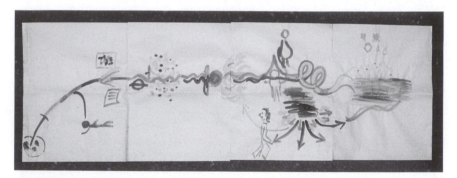

Figure 5.8   Lifeline: Marian
Source: Photograph by David Newton

We slightly overran our time and had to hurry the discussion, so that we did not spend as long on the last few paintings as we would have liked. Everyone seemed to have enjoyed the session and one or two in particular seemed to have gained a lot from it. We certainly got to know each other and our lives in a way we had not done before, and this helped us to understand each other better. This exercise also seemed to give people a sense of perspective by enabling them to stand back and look at their lives as a whole.

Group painting

On another occasion when Heather was away, there were only four of us there and the atmosphere seemed quite flat and low. I made various sugges-tions, most of which did not seem to appeal. Finally, the idea of doing a group painting seemed to raise enthusiasm (Figure 5.9). To start, we closed our eyes and with charcoal 'took a line for a walk' for a few minutes, then opened our eyes to look. In silence, we painted using our 'squiggle' as a basis to turn into anything that suggested itself. Then we moved out to meet the others and carried on until we had covered the paper, which took nearly an hour. Two of us painted much faster than the others, so that at times we seemed to be in danger of swamping them. The finished result still showed clearly the four contributions, which were as follows.

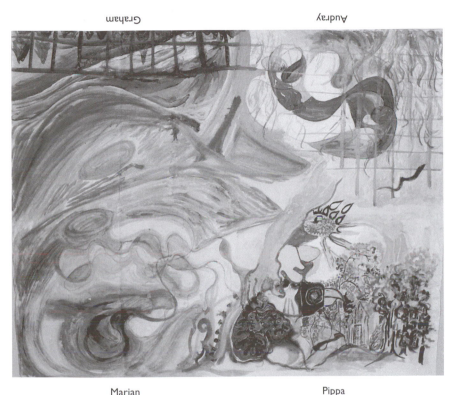

Graham   Audray

Marian   Pippa

Figure 5.9   Group painting by four members of the 'Friday Group'
Source: Photograph by David Newton

Myself (bottom left)

Abstract swirls of yellow, orange, red, blue and green, with an intense blue shape emerging in the centre.

Pippa (bottom right)

On the far right, she had started by painting a nostalgic scene of the house and garden her family had left a year previously, and which she had loved. She had painted the sun in because children often do, and she still sometimes felt very much a child. Then, without quite meaning to, she had painted two aborted foetuses (bottom left) being plucked out by a long, muscular arm reaching down from above. She had in fact had two abortions – one some years back and the other one only the previous week – and was still trying to clear her mind about it. She had not meant to tell anyone – the foetuses just 'popped up' in the painting. Her doctor had been against the abortion, but as she and her husband already had three children she felt they had made the right decision. We spent quite a while in the group discussing it and I encouraged her to carry on using painting to 'clear her mind'.

Audrey (top right, but described from her way up)

She started by filling in the charcoal curves with red, blue and purple, then felt some straight lines were needed to balance these and painted grey criss-cross lines, which she said were prison bars representing her husband and her marriage. The flames at the bottom left were the fire she was looking for inside herself – but at the same time she was frightened, in case the fire led to an explosion. She did not want her marriage to break up. When someone asked her about the dark blue bird hovering above, Audrey burst into tears and said it was herself wishing to 'fly' but feeling she couldn't.

Graham (top left, but described from his way up)

He started with browns and greens near the bottom, then widened out and mirrored my sweeps of colour and egg shape. Then he added strong splodges of red (centre) and finally a fence which echoed Audrey's prison bars, and a few trees to make a 'Swiss landscape' (although he had never been to Switzerland).

For most of the group it was their first experience of doing a group painting, which probably accounts for the fact that the individual contributions are mostly fairly separate. It can be quite a threatening experience, in a culture which stresses individuality, to suddenly try to merge with others in doing a group painting. The whole morning was a very deep and moving shared experience for all of us and it was quite difficult for us to clear up and go home.

Melting mirror

This was a fantasy journey led by Heather in which we imagined we were standing in front of a mirror, which then melted and shook, leaving us face to face with ourselves as children in a room we knew well and liked. What was that child saying to us and what would our reply be? As we gathered up our paints, it turned out that all of us were 'stuck' as we needed more time to 'get into it', so we asked Heather to go through it again. The resulting paintings looked at ourselves at different ages and places. Here are a few examples.

Ruth

Ruth's picture showed her taking a photograph of herself, aged three or four, dressed up as a queen, in her back garden where she spent most of her time playing on her own. She had not had a very happy childhood and this was her escape. The following week, Ruth reported that the image she had painted of herself had haunted her during the week and she had felt rather stirred up by it.

Jenny

Jenny's main memory was of some very special pink-flowered wallpaper and the brown lino that was prevalent at the time. This rang bells with several other members of the group whose memories were also coloured by ubiquitous brown lino.

Pippa

Pippa was facing the same way as herself, looking out of the picture in her favourite room – her grandparents' bathroom in Denmark. There was a long arm dropping her on the floor, and the message of the picture seemed to be that she felt she had not fulfilled her early promise.

Myself

I was talking to my 8-year-old self who was saying 'Come and play outside' in my favourite childhood haunts of old logs and bracken near our house. This too seemed to be an escape from other things in life that were difficult.

Venetia

Venetia was an art therapist with three grown-up children and had just joined the group on moving to Bristol. In her mirror she was about 12, tall and slim, in a white tennis outfit, in her new room, and wanting very much to be grown up. Now, as her adult self, she felt much more able to appreciate her childlike traits, so there was an interesting reversal going on.

Once again we realised how much our child selves were still parts of our current selves. This exercise helped us to get a dialogue going between our child and adult selves and alerted us to needs we still had, but often ignored. It was also a chance to appreciate the positive qualities of our child selves and to integrate these into our adult lives.

In between these sessions, Heather was asking the group to interpret some of Kelly's theories in paint. For example, aggression as 'expanding boundaries' compared with hostility as 'defensive action'; and guilt as 'discovering you were not the person you thought you were'. We explored these in pictures and discussed them.

Towards Easter we knew we needed to discuss with the group whether it should continue into the summer. Both Heather and I decided that we needed a six-week break because of other commitments. We discussed the starting date of the next term and discovered that several people were very disappointed at the idea of such a long break. Our final session before the break was a group mural, which shows some of these feelings.

Group mural

We all joined in the mural, painting wherever we wanted (Figures 5.10 and 5.11). Figure 5.10 shows the group at work, and Figure 5.11 the finished mural. We were using liquid ready-mixed thick paint. On the left, Graham's contribution – very distinct and full of esoteric symbols – has a face underground 'pushing up the daisies'. The £40K? referred to the 'price on that person's head', he said. He drew a line to keep his patch separate. Moving towards the right, the blazing sun and grassy bonfire were mine, also some small solid flowers underneath the fire. The tall slender flowering plant was Heather's, as were the birds high in the sky. Jenny did a blue shape full of £ signs (money worries) surrounded by heavy black and red lines. Audrey placed herself on the edge and painted a very solid green house (bottom right). Ruth was working at the top right on cloud formations, stimulated by an earlier discussion with Jenny on Steiner's use of peach colour. In between the peach-coloured clouds Ruth included blue triangles, which she blended into boomerang shapes to link with Heather's birds. She wanted to 'flow' into Audrey's space, but the hard edge of the house was intimidating and she was afraid of offending Audrey. It was interesting to see that later Audrey herself continued Ruth's swirls by making her own dark flowing strokes across her house. Ruth also tried to link Graham's section with the whole of the mural, but Graham quickly reaffirmed his position by going over the line separating his part from the rest. Right at the end, Heather decided to add some insects and a 'can of worms' at the bottom of the picture, seen by others as a touch of 'reality'.

During the discussion afterwards, it came out that Jenny's blue, black and red shape was a mixture of depression and anger at the long break. Several people echoed this, saying how much the group meant to them and how it was their 'safe space' which was just theirs. Instances were

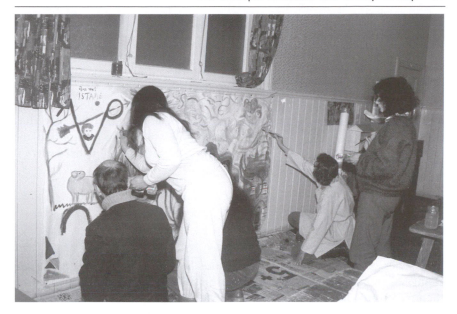

Figure 5.10 The 'Friday Group' at work on a mural
Source: Photograph by Heather Buddery

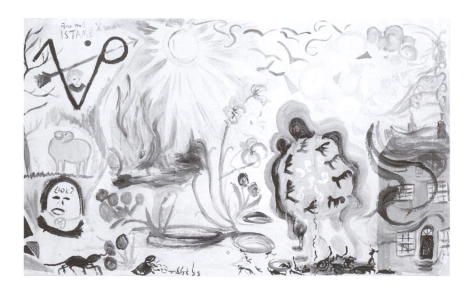

Figure 5.11 Group mural by the 'Friday Group'
Source: Photograph by David Newton

mentioned when this 'safe space' had been spoilt or violated. Some members of the group decided to meet socially halfway through the break, to help them over the time when they would be missing the weekly sessions. Obviously when the new term started its length and purpose would need to be discussed.

The group mural brought us together as a group, while allowing everyone to portray their individual concerns. The positions taken up by different people demonstrated how they saw themselves in the group, and the interactions on paper showed the group process at work. In these ways it proved a fitting ritual to end the term.

Conclusion

This series of group sessions demonstrates how the nature of a group can change. The group members came together as a class and developed into a therapy group, by everyone's consent. Although no one was deemed to need the intervention of an institution, most people were at that moment carrying problems of some magnitude (divorce, long-term unemployment, depression, marriage problems, work problems, mental illness, big decisions, etc.) which they were trying to sort out in their own way. In many ways the problems shared were a typical cross-section of those around in the community at large, and the usefulness of art therapy in the group shows how widely applicable it can be. Heather's open approach and the freedom to come and go were most important to group members (although in fact attendance was very regular).

This account may seem somewhat disjointed because it is impossible, within the space of a chapter, to give a real idea of an ongoing group and the sharing of personal lives entailed. It is not an example of a 'perfect' group – rather the ups and downs of an experimental community group exploring themselves through personal painting and discussion. The final word comes from Ruth, one of the group members, writing just before the Easter break:

> Looking back over the weeks, there seems to be a good deal of significance in the work done on Fridays. I have been working on a large-scale painting at home which begins to link images from the past and from the Friday group. It appears to be a picking-up of stitches and knitting together to find a wholeness and continuity in my life. I am the creator of my life, and the pattern changes as external events or internal conflicts cause me to falter or change direction. Now I am better able to see the pattern of the past, and maybe even the shape of things to come.

References

Burr, V. and Butt, T. (1992) *Invitation to Personal Construct Psychology*, London: Whurr.

Dalton, P. and Dunnett, G. (1999) *A Psychology for Living: Personal Construct Theory for Professionals and Clients*, Preston: ECPA.

Fransella, F. (1995) *George Kelly (Key Figures in Counselling and Psychotherapy)*, London: Sage.

Kelly, G. (1963) *A Theory of Personality: The Psychology of Personal Constructs*, New York: Norton.

Chapter 6

Examples of groups

In this chapter I shall give some more examples of art therapy and personal art groups in a variety of settings. This is not a typical or a comprehensive selection, but gives an indication of the range of possibilities. The accounts are necessarily subjective, from the point of view of the therapist or facilitator. This chapter is not designed to be read in one sitting, but rather to be used as a compendium to browse in, according to your particular interest. The chapter is divided as follows (the themes used are included in italics):

Residential institutions
1 Admission ward in a large urban psychiatric hospital (*Past, present and future*)
2 Groupwork with clients with learning disabilities (*Group murals*)
3 Small therapeutic centre in the country (*Clay trees representing selves*)
4 Young women with eating disorders (*'I wonder' wall*)

Psychiatric day patients/clients
5 Day hospital group looking at family emotions (*Painting on wet paper, How people experienced their parents sorting out conflicts*)
6 Day hospital 'stuck' group (*How see self, how others see you, how like to be*)
7 Anger management art therapy group in a community mental health team (*Anger themes*)
8 Long-term community support group (*Spiral lifeline, Practical group project, Winter colours, Community of selves*)

Specialised day hospitals and centres
9 Day hospital for older adults (*Initials design, Weddings*)
10 Alcohol unit (*Masks of others and self, Body outlines, Group painting*)
11 Day centre for ex-offenders (*Metaphorical portraits*)
12 Cancer help centre (*Guided imagery of journey under the sea*)
13 Children experiencing difficulties (*Family tree, Exploring silence*)
14 Asian women's group (*Anger and family issues*)

Staff groups
15 Residential children's workers (*Group painting, Family tree*)
16 Staff at a day hospital for older adults (*How see self, how others see you – professionally*)
17 Art therapy option on counselling skills course (*Building a community, Self boxes*)
18 Teachers of peace education (*Introduction pictures, Conversation in pairs, Group painting*)
19 Workshop for mediators on 'Art and Conflict' (*Sharing space, Visual mediation*)
20 Race and culture workshops for art therapists (*Image of racist, Cultural identity*)

Community situations
21 'Art as Communication' day workshop (*Introduction pictures, Conversation in pairs, Round Robin drawings, Group mandala, Metaphorical portraits*)
22 Women's group (*Current feelings, Round Robin drawings, Group picture*)
23 Workshop for second generation Jewish group (*Introduction pictures, Exploring heritage*)
24 Mixed group of adults and children (*Transport collages*)

The following describe one session in an ongoing series: 1, 3, 4, 5, 6, 9, 11, 13.

The following describe briefly a whole series of sessions: 2, 7, 8, 10, 14, 17.

The following describe single-occasion groups: 12, 15, 16, 18, 19, 20, 21, 22, 23, 24.

Residential institutions

1. Admission ward in a large urban psychiatric hospital

This was one of a regular series for patients on an acute admissions ward in a large psychiatric hospital. There were five patients on this occasion, mostly people who had been in an art therapy group before, and well known to the art therapist, Sheena. The patients included one person with a long-standing alcohol problem, another suffering from agoraphobia and three others whose diagnosis Sheena did not know. Three were women and two were men. There were also four members of staff: herself, an art therapy student (a woman), an occupational therapy student (a woman) and a medical student (a man).

It always took a while to get a group together on an admission ward because the patients were in a fairly bad way and found it difficult both to motivate themselves to get there and to function well in the group once they had arrived. The group took place in the occupational therapy room attached to the ward. It was large and quiet, with pleasant posters on the wall, and had a group of tables with chairs round it on one side and a circle of easychairs on the other side.

Sheena welcomed everyone and asked people to say their names and one or two words about how they were feeling. Then she asked them to spend 10 to 15 minutes drawing or painting anything they liked. There were plenty of materials to hand, and most people used paints, with a couple preferring crayons. While they were finishing, Sheena made some coffee to help the atmosphere to be informal and sociable.

After coffee, she introduced the main theme: past, present and future, all on one piece of paper. She reassured people by saying that although looking into the future could be quite 'scary', it could be a good thing to do in a safe environment.

Most people divided their paper into three with lines and worked for quite a long time. When most people had finished, the group moved on to discussion. Sheena asked everyone to look back to their first paintings, and each person in turn talked about both paintings she/he had done. There was not time to talk about everything, so she made sure that at least all the patients had a chance to say what they wanted.

In general, most of the patients saw their past as wonderful, a state to 'get back to'. They saw their present as muddled, confused and unhappy and their future as fairly bleak and hopeless. By contrast, most of the staff members' futures were much more optimistic. Some examples will clarify this.

Margaret

Her past showed a nice house and a nice husband, and she saw the past as totally rosy. Her present was empty, save for some black clouds. Her future consisted of some grey land together with some grey and black birds. Sheena asked her if a change of colour would lead to a more hopeful outlook and Margaret said, 'I suppose it could do. When I feel a bit better, I expect I'll see the future as more hopeful.'

Raymond

His introductory painting depicted a lone cottage with a red roof, in open countryside – a wish he had always had as a child and had never been able to fulfil (his present accommodation, on his own, was in a block of flats). His past showed him with his wife, together with his four sons and their girlfriends, drawn as stick figures in pink and green, all happy. His present showed himself, and – in a box laid on its side – his dead wife. His future showed himself in pink in a box lying on its side (i.e. dead), all the sons in green, their spouses in black, and then rows and rows of red figures, all the future children. This fitted in with his interpretation of the future as 'carrying on the bloodstock'. He said it was not up to him to 'tamper with fate', and the general feeling emanating from his pictures was that he felt he had no power to change his life.

Medical student

For his 'present' he drew himself with huge, outstretched arms like a giant Christ, stethoscope round his neck, filling most of the available space, above a sea of tiny coloured people. When others asked who the tiny people were, he said they were his friends on the course. The group did not quite believe him. They had a sneaking suspicion that they were patients, as the picture portrayed very accurately the enormous power they felt doctors had over patients.

Sheena

Sheena always liked to join in, as she felt that the group went better if she did. Her past showed a heavy panelled door with a brass knob. The door was shut – she felt one could never go back. Her image of the present was herself juggling with several coloured balls, precariously keeping everything going. Life was hectic, but pretty good. Her future showed her firmly on her feet, arms outstretched holding two golden balls, looking happy. When she looked at it again in the discussion time, she and others all thought perhaps it looked a bit static and her 'present' looked more interesting and lively.

The discussion was curtailed by an over-efficient nurse, who telephoned the room ten minutes early to see if they were ready for lunch. As soon as lunch was mentioned, everyone rushed off – leaving Sheena to clear up.

This group shows the bleakness felt by many inpatients in psychiatric hospitals and the theme used had enabled group members to express this, as well as trying to set their problems in perspective by looking backward and forward.

2. Groupwork with clients with learning disabilities

This was a group for eight male clients with moderate learning difficulties, who had been living in a hospital for most of their lives and were institutionalised. They were of varying ages between 22 and 72 and were fairly articulate. They all had some form of 'challenging behaviour', such as aggression or violence, usually as a reaction to specific situations. For instance, one or two of them would hit out or smash objects on the ward if asked to do certain things.

The treatments and activities included medication, behaviour modification, occupational therapy and industrial therapy. The art therapy group was introduced to help them learn to express their feelings in a more appropriate way, and learn to 'self-advocate' in an acceptable manner. Richard, the therapist, decided to do a series of groupwork sessions using large paper pinned on the wall. For the first session he used eight A1 sheets on the wall, and emptied the room of everything except a semi-circle of chairs. He gave the group slightly different structures to work with each week, such as:

- Ask people to take turns making marks on the paper. This was a fairly controlled process but also quite exposing for individuals.
- Leave it to the group. It was always interesting to see who went first, who formed partnerships with others. Sometimes everyone allocated themselves to a sheet of paper each.
- Ask people to move around.
- Ask people to work in pairs.
- Number the sheets and make a group journey from sheet one to sheet eight.
- Ask people to work in two groups. It was then interesting to see whether groups took up themes of the other group or just obliterated them.

There was an infinite number of variations, using different shapes and sizes of paper, and different themes. Materials could be varied too. On occasions Richard suggested the group worked on the floor. This had a different dynamic. Whereas clients could see the wall picture all the time while contributing to it, on the floor it was hard to see what was happening as a whole while working on one part. But it was also possible to use messier materials on the floor.

Richard encouraged the group to interact, talk, discuss, negotiate with each other, as these were skills to be learnt and practised. Occasionally, for the contrast and to work on non-verbal skills, he asked them to work in silence.

The men attended the group for varying lengths of time from one to five years. During their time in the group, several clients learnt to speak for themselves and left the hospital for a community setting. Others took longer. Although the group had been set up to help clients make these moves, in some ways it was working against the prevailing ethos of the ward, which had been set up as a place for people who would always be disabled and needed looking after. The group also brought out feelings of group members of being deprived of 'normality', a frequent theme for people with learning disabilities.

This example shows how different themes and structures for groupwork can generate different dynamics and results. It also shows how groupwork can be used for a group of moderately learning disabled men to find their voice and begin to shape their own futures.

3. Small therapeutic centre in the country

This therapeutic centre was situated in an old manor house in beautiful countryside and had accommodation for about 10 to 12 persons. The patients were mostly between the ages of 18 to 25 years and were referred there by doctors or other caring professionals. As the centre had gained official recognition, the patients were able to get their treatment costs and expenses paid. Most of them were depressed, but not ill enough to be taken into a psychiatric hospital. Some had a history of drug problems.

There were daily therapy sessions, both group and individual, and the patients took part in the general running of the centre, doing gardening and maintenance work, helping to prepare meals and so on. The art therapy sessions took place once a week in the afternoon, after a long group therapy session, which sometimes ended late.

This particular session took place outside in the courtyard, as it was a beautiful warm sunny day. Clay was used instead of the more usual paint. There were five patients and an art therapy trainee, as well as the art therapist, Linnea. She asked everyone to model a tree out of clay to represent themselves, adding any other available natural materials such as stones, sticks and leaves, if they wished. When the trees were finished, Linnea asked people to place them on a large piece of plywood to create a 'forest'.

When the group sculpture was finished, it was easy to see that each tree was an individual expression of its creator. Some had outstretched hands as branches, others had unstable trunks and lacked a solid base. One was surrounded by an impenetrable ring of stones, another scarcely visible under a heavy blanket of leaves. Here and there, paths leading to neighbouring trees indicated responses to others.

One person, Dan, didn't make a clay tree at all. He made a clay mountain at one end of the board and then stuck wind-blown 'stick' trees at the top and painted a blue river running down the side towards the other trees, to water them. Finally, he modelled a house on stilts, with a ladder leading up to it, and placed it by the river. His whole contribution was very beautiful, and others made paths from their trees to his 'protecting' mountain and welcoming house. This very much represented Dan who, despite his own problems of isolation and depression, spent a lot of time looking after others. He had a quiet, solid interior that drew others to him.

It was a very successful and enjoyable session, and all the more so because it led to a deep discussion of feelings about where people felt they were, both on the plywood board and in the rest of their lives.

4. Young women with eating disorders

The 'I Wonder' Wall: a tool to build a bridge from silence to voice

This art therapy group took place in a residential unit for young women aged 16 to 19 with long-term chronic eating disorders. The aim of the group was to help them express their feelings, but they were initially very resistant to anything that might be about 'therapy', which implied the suggestion that they might contemplate some change. The art therapist, Nicky, usually worked non-directively but recognised the need to provide some exercises at the beginning to encourage the young women to use the therapeutic space.

So Nicky started by introducing different ways of using the art media, such as making permanent marks on paper, choosing colours of paint and squirting them onto thick paper, passing images round for everyone to contribute to them, 'consequences' with pictures, and so on. All these were aimed at helping the young women to feel safer with the media and with the space. At various times Nicky would ask 'I wonder what people are feeling today/about this activity?' but often she was met with what she felt as a stony, even persecutory silence. The young women would not talk to each other in the groups very much either.

One day, about three months after the start of the sessions, one young woman (Carly) who had been particularly 'anti-therapy', came in with a present for Nicky. It was Carly's way of accepting and appreciating staff she liked without having to say so directly. The present was a T-shirt on which she had carefully painted the words 'I WONDER HOW THE REST OF THE GROUP FEEL ABOUT ME WEARING THIS T-SHIRT' (see Figure 6.1). Carly's idea was for Nicky to wear the T-shirt bearing the words 'I wonder . . .' which Carly saw as Nicky's trademark 'therapist-speak'.

The T-shirt was actually too small for Nicky (people with eating disorders often have problems with accurate perception of size) but it gave her an idea. The next week she brought in the T-shirt on a tailor's dummy and also about 100 small cut-out paper T-shirts, varying in size from thumb-size up to A4. At the end of the room she had covered one wall with hardboard and labelled it the 'I-WONDER' WALL. She asked the group members to select any of the paper T-shirt shapes and write a question beginning 'I wonder . . .'. For instance: 'I wonder why it's so quiet in here?' 'I wonder what it's like for staff in this group?', and so on. These would then be pinned anonymously on the 'I-wonder' wall. At this stage in the group there were always two other consistent staff present and four young women in the group.

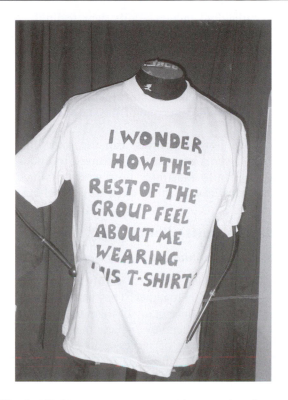

Figure 6.1   'I Wonder' T-shirt – young women with eating disorders
Source: Photograph by Nicky Linfield

At first no one moved. Then one person reached out for a tiny T-shirt shape, then another, until all were busy in their own safe spaces around the room. They put their T-shirt messages on the wall, or other members of the group did so. Some of the young women cut out their own T-shirt shapes of varying sizes. Soon the wall was full of T-shirts with 'I wonder' questions and statements, and the activity stopped when the group energy waned. Then everyone read the messages and began to talk about them – what they felt about what they saw, and how they had felt writing about others. Some of the questions were:

- I wonder if Nicky gets frustrated?
- I wonder what is the point in doing this?
- I wonder how it will be with new people joining the group?

There were also personal wonderings about each other. The exercise gave rise to quite a bit of laughter about some of the comments. Finally group members created individual images about their feelings. They seemed to have found a new freedom to do this.

This session opened the door to some honest communication and seemed to give permission for the young women to voice their views. It helped even the most resistant participants to join in the group and find a creative process they could use. Carly, whose 'anti-therapy' T-shirt was the original inspiration for the session, became one of the stalwarts who used the group to its full potential.

This example shows how a therapist can use something that has happened in the group – even a provocative gesture – to find a theme to bring the group together. It also illustrates how writing (which is often quite private) and visual work can be interwoven to good effect.

Psychiatric day patients/clients

5. Day hospital group looking at family emotions

This was a new group of eight patients, mostly suffering from depression, who all happened to be starting together. They had not done any art therapy before and it was a long time since many of them had used art materials. The art therapist, Roy, wanted them to bypass the usual inhibitions about 'producing art' and feel a sense of success and excitement from using art materials in a new way. So he suggested that group members should wet their paper, choose a few colours they liked and play around, being aware of their feelings about the colours and shapes produced. Then, if their painting seemed to suggest a definite pattern or image to them, they could develop this image further pictorially if they wished. The results were very varied:

- One picture, mostly yellow, had a thick line across it. How did that person feel about it? It transpired that she felt she had to keep her feelings bottled in.
- A painting of cheerful flowers on a black table turned out to be related to the brave front that person was trying to keep up.
- A rich picture with a desert, fertile places and a waterfall in the foreground seemed to be linked with feelings and emotions pouring out, irrigating an otherwise barren world.

As people shared their pictures, there seemed to be many unresolved conflicts, bottled-up feelings and simmering emotions, many of them connected with marriage problems. At home, these led to anger and rows and misgivings as to whether these were justified. When the group members met the next week they discussed all these things and Roy suggested the theme: how they had experienced their parents sorting out their conflicts.

The results of these were illuminating. One woman, Shirley, remembered her father being very passive and 'saintly', and not able to cope with any emotion. Her mother had lost a child and got so distraught grieving over this on her own that she was considered mentally ill. Shirley had never shared this with anyone and now saw herself as being like her mother, and her own husband cool and saintly like her father. She was frightened at her own anger, and concluded that she too must be crazy.

Another woman identified with this. Morag felt that she could not get through to her husband, despite making wilder and wilder efforts. He was seen as a 'pillar of the community' and she felt her anger must therefore be unacceptable. She had painted herself as a glass cage with horrible things on show inside.

The shared pictures and feelings meant that, for the first time, these women felt they were not alone. The rest of the group also said they felt it was normal to be angry in this situation. Many tears were shed that session and the two women felt at last that they were acceptable.

Roy felt that the next step might be to explore ways they might change their situations. After discussion the next week, he thought an enabling theme could be: 'What do you fear might happen if you let out your bottled-up feelings?' or 'How would you like to behave at home?' or 'What is frustrating you at the moment?' Usually people had three fears:

- They might destroy others.
- They might destroy themselves.
- Nothing at all might happen.

Roy felt these themes were very powerful and produced a strong reaction in the group, but he also felt that if people were experiencing these feelings, it was right to suggest a theme that would facilitate their expression. A 'tea-and-sympathy' approach which ignored this would only reinforce their misgivings about having these very feelings. After all, that was the reason people were attending the day hospital. As an experienced art therapist, he felt reasonably confident in handling strong emotions, and there was further support for the patients at the day hospital from nurses and doctors. He encouraged people to open up, at the same time making it clear that people did not have to expose themselves emotionally if they did not wish to.

This account shows the use of the group, both in checking out each other's perceptions and in providing support for each other. The themes were chosen to fit into this process and maximise the benefits of being part of such a group.

6. Day hospital 'stuck' group

Not all art sessions give rise to interesting discussion full of insights which promote personal change. Some groups are so 'stuck' that they remain caught in the same old patterns whatever is tried. The session described below is one of these. It took place at a day hospital attached to a large psychiatric hospital. Patients came to the day hospital daily for six to eight weeks, for a programme of art therapy, psychodrama, psychotherapy, yoga, discussion groups, etc.

On this particular occasion the group comprised the art therapist, John, and six patients (two men, four women), one aged 20, three in their forties and two in their fifties. The older ones were suffering from a cluster of problems, such as chronic marriage problems, children leaving home, long-term unemployment, phobias, etc., while the one younger woman had problems with parents and boyfriends. John described the group members as 'casualties of society', for whom there was little hope, especially in the social climate at that point. Change was very difficult for them, especially as they got older. Society in general seemed to be offering fewer options to those finding life difficult and John sometimes tried to cultivate an awareness of these perspectives.

This group had been working together for some weeks and was about to finish its programme in a further week. So John chose a theme (in consultation with the day hospital team) related to the outside world and their future aspirations. He always started with a 'warm-up' in which he asked people to paint how they were feeling and, if possible, to include themselves in the picture. Then, for the main theme, he asked them to do a picture containing:

(a) how you see yourself
(b) how others see you, maybe someone close to you
(c) how you would like to be.

Everyone worked away for about half an hour, using oil pastels (John had to carry all the art materials from the art therapy room to the day hospital). The rest of the time was spent in discussion and looking at the pictures. It would take too long to describe everyone's work so I have chosen two of the group and will describe their pictures.

Molly

Molly was in her early forties and had been an in-patient. She was anxious and depressed and felt her family didn't care about her – only looked to her to service their needs (meals, washing-up, etc.).

WARM-UP

Chaotic picture of the confusion in Molly's mind, which she felt she could not share with her family because they were sick of hearing it. She also had death on her mind a lot (her own).

THEME

(a) She saw herself as boring and black (she was a black woman and had experienced racism on account of this when she was at school).
(b) She showed herself wearing a 'nice' mask, which she had worn for a long time when she worked as a domestic. Sadly, this mask was now broken.
(c) She had not been able to do this part. She just did not know how she would like to be.

Jim

Jim was in his early fifties, divorced, and had been made redundant from his job as a sales rep. When he was working, his social life had revolved around the drinking connected with his job. Now he was very lonely and was disliked by the women staff at the day hospital because he was so lecherous.

WARM-UP

A picture of a maze, which he related to his attempts to find a job.

THEME

(a) A thick black vertical band, with a thin yellow one to the right of it. He said this was about his depression and unemployment.
(b) The same as (a). He seemed to have no idea about the effect he had on other people, or the way the hospital staff saw him.
(c) He drew more vertical lines and bands of colour, but these were more brightly coloured – blue, yellow, red, orange. He wanted to be confident, independent and working, with a car, social life and friends. All his hopes for himself were bound up with work, although his chances of finding any were negligible during the recession at that time.

John felt very frustrated with the outcome of this group because he felt that most of its members were the victims of oppressions not in his power to alleviate – such as racism, sexism and women's roles, unemployment, lack of education. All he felt he could do was to help them realise that the state they were in was not totally their fault, and hope that this awareness would lift a corner of their misery and enable small changes in their attitudes towards themselves.

7. Anger management art therapy group in a community mental health team

A male community psychiatric nurse and I facilitated this art therapy group, to help people with mental health problems who were having difficulty coping with anger. It was designed as an opportunity for people to look at ways of managing anger, so that it was less destructive to themselves and others. Each session included artwork and sharing and finished with relaxation. Members of the group were expected to attend all the sessions. The programme covered the following:

1 Introductions and ground rules.
2 Relaxation and guided imagery.
3 What is anger?
4 Physical symptoms of anger. Anger – good or bad?
5 What's underneath the anger?
6 Early family patterns.
7 Anger and conflict.
8 Feelings and assertiveness, I-messages.
9 Picture review.
10 Group picture and ending.

Art therapy has several particular things to offer in work on anger management:

(a) It helps people who find it hard to articulate verbally why they get angry.
(b) The process of doing the artwork slows them down and helps them to reflect more on what is going on.
(c) Sharing the artwork helps people realise that they have things in common with each other and overcomes isolation.
(d) Doing artwork enables a group to include both those who 'act out' their anger on others and those who 'act in' their anger on themselves (in a verbal group it is often difficult to include both of these in the same group).

Formulating ground rules was particularly important in making the group a safe place to work on a subject often seen as frightening, so we spent half a session on it, including everyone's suggestions. For the same reason the relaxation was important – both to teach it as a method to help with anger and as a way of letting go of any upsetting feelings at the end of a session. Several different forms of relaxation were used, together with guided imagery (e.g. a favourite peaceful place), and members showed an increasing ability to use it in the sessions and in their lives.

Handouts were available for all the different aspects of anger management. Some people found these useful, some not. Several clients asked for sets to be sent to their key workers after the group.

Referrals and attendance

Referrals came from all parts of the mental health team and applicants were asked to attend an informal interview to check commitment and suitability (from our own and the client's point of view), and to help prepare them for the group. In the inner city mental health service, attendance was always a problem. Of the 17 referrals, 8 clients actually started the group and 4 dropped out along the way, for a variety of reasons. There seemed to be a gender issue, as the group that finished consisted of three men and one woman, who then left because she found the group 'too male orientated'. However, she was persuaded to return to explain her reasons.

We asked everyone to write down before their interview how they saw their problems with anger. Their answers included such things as:

- If things go wrong, I get angry and lose my temper.
- I get stressed and wound up in lots of situations, leading to anger.
- I cannot handle family situations.
- I have to be on my guard all the time.
- Punching walls and windows.
- Violence to other people.

The group

The group developed well from a cautious start. The participants started to find links between each other and relaxed a bit. With each session, group members found it easier to get involved in the artwork, which then gave rise to interesting discussion.

The fourth session included a look at the physical symptoms of anger, which we drew on an outline of a body (see Figure 6.2). The resulting composite image showed the cumulative effects of anger, and was useful in helping participants become aware of their own anger and that of others. One man, Dave, disclosed for the first time a lump in his throat (depicted as a round red blob with arrows radiating from it) when he felt angry, and was surprised to find he was not on his own. Over the course of the rest of the sessions, this lump disappeared for him. He also contributed the wavy line for the mouth, which he described as an 'angry sneer'.

In the fifth session, people found it quite hard to look at some of the emotions underlying their anger – sadness and illness featured here, but people found it hard to express these. The same was true for the sixth session, on family patterns, which unsurprisingly was an emotional session.

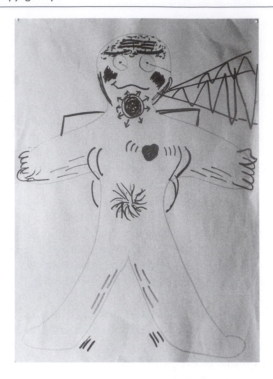

Figure 6.2 Physical symptoms of anger – anger management art therapy group
Source: Photograph by Anna Coldham

The seventh session looked at the negative and positive messages in people's heads and how these can 'wind people up' or help to calm them down. Dave's picture (Figure 6.3) showed how far he had come. It related to an incident the previous week at the mental health day hospital he attended when 'someone started on him'. The left-hand side of the picture showed his habitual way of responding – to retaliate in a heavy way, carrying it on into a feud lasting 'hours, days, weeks, months', in 'ever-decreasing circles'. The right-hand side showed how he thought about it for a moment, then decided to keep a 'healthy distance' between him and the other person and not respond. He discovered that this only took minutes to clear up and left him feeling a happier person. The 'problems buried' referred to his sense of control in deciding not to allow someone else's behaviour to become a problem for him.

In the eighth session, on assertiveness, the artwork focused on 'the real you'. This was preceded by an initial round about 'a time I felt good about myself', which showed that this was a very rare experience for the three men present at that session. In one case the only occasion had been 30 years previously. Again, it was an emotive session.

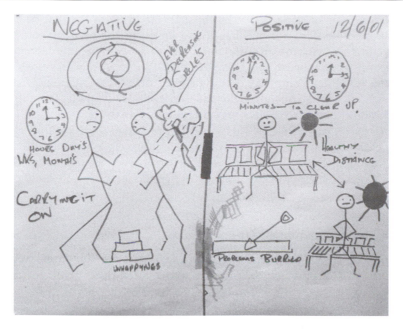

Figure 6.3   Anger and conflict: negative and positive messages – anger management art therapy group
Source: Photograph by Anna Coldham

The ninth session was a review of the pictures done during the first eight sessions (which had been kept in folders in the art therapy room), followed by a picture on an important aspect summing things up. The final session, rounding things off, was a group exercise on 'Gifts' in which everyone drew metaphorical gifts in each other's boxes and baskets. One man was so touched he was nearly in tears, going home clutching his gift picture carefully.

Evaluation

The evaluation questionnaires and post-group interviews provided an opportunity for reflection on what participants had learnt, and also for a handover to the professionals who would be continuing to work with group members. Group members had particularly valued the opportunity for artwork, meeting others with similar problems and the honest discussions.

Dave had found the group hard but attended every week. His earlier pictures were all outline drawings in one colour felt-tip pen, but as he made progress in the later sessions he introduced more colours and his drawings were more creative. He was very talkative – in fact unable to stop on several occasions. Initially he found the relaxation very difficult, but was much more able to settle into it by the end. He came to see that he could tolerate others different from himself and let go of the need to 'sort them out', getting on with his own life more. As a result he became less intimidating and more relaxed and open. He was able to deal with upsets in a different, less threatening way. Other people noticed the difference. At the end he said it was the first group he had ever completed and he found doing the relaxation and the pictures very useful.

The anger management art therapy group provided a vehicle for helping a few clients to make significant changes in the way they handled their anger and expressed themselves. The artwork and the relaxation were both important factors in this, as was the group support and building of relationships.

8. Long-term community support group

This group of about ten men and women, aged 30 to 60, met once a week at the local day hospital for long-term support after their treatment as an inpatient or day patient had finished. They were mostly living in bedsitters and unemployed and felt pretty lonely and isolated. Heather, the art therapist, saw the purpose of the weekly art therapy session as mainly supportive, to provide some social contact and stimulate the interest of group members. She decided to focus on the world around, especially the natural world, to help them to be more aware of their surroundings and opportunities available. Heather tried to introduce all the activities in such a way that members of the group could relate to them in small everyday ways. This helped them to make a start and also to keep their experiences relevant to their lives. The following series describes the different ways in which she used this broad theme over a period of several weeks.

Spiral lifeline

This was an introductory session, to help Heather to get to know the group, and to help group members to get to know each other. To warm up, she introduced the idea of spirals and the group thought of examples in nature such as corkscrews, whirlwinds, etc. Then they drew quick spirals on paper, moving on to a big spiral starting from birth, which they developed to show important events in their lives. Heather also asked them to extend the spiral into the future, to remind them that their lives did not stop at the present.

Practical group project

To help the group members feel more at ease with each other, Heather introduced a simple group project in which everyone could join. It was winter, with thick snow, and birds could not find food. Members of the group spent a long time carefully making little bird cakes for the many birds in the day hospital grounds. The proud moment came when they went outside, placed the cakes on the birdtable and waited to see if the birds would eat them. The day hospital was situated right next to the sea, and before the land birds could reach the cakes a crowd of large, greedy seagulls swooped down and gobbled them all up. This rapid demolition of their hard work gave the group members a lesson about nature that they had not been expecting, but fortunately they were able to see the funny side.

Winter colours

As late winter was a particularly difficult and dreary time for people eking out lives in cold bedsitters, Heather wanted to see if she could mobilise group members' imaginations to bring more colour into their world. She often felt that for many people colour was more evocative and immediate than shape, so she liked to start sessions with an experience based on pure colour.

On this occasion, Heather asked people to think what colour they would associate with February. After that, she asked people to imagine what each of their five senses would suggest for February, and relate this to themselves in some kind of poem or picture. The pictures were all very different, showing the variety of associations with February.

Although people's initial reactions to February had been 'How dull!', they soon found a variety of colours and associations. Some chose browns and greys, while others remembered that snowdrops and celandines made their appearance then, and added whites and delicate yellows. Someone else thought of the purple of buds preparing themselves for spring, while 'indoor types' built up fires of oranges and reds.

Community of selves

Heather asked people to think of all their different roles and 'selves', e.g. mother/son/housewife/car driver, etc., and to draw them all together as a community. She saw this theme as a way of helping group members to value the roles and skills they did have, at a time when the 'outside world' gave them little recognition. It surprised people how many different roles they could think of for themselves. They also jogged each other's memories as they realised others' roles applied to them too. This in turn engendered a good spirit in the group and a feeling of optimism.

Over the weeks, as group members shared experiences and worked together, they seemed to take more interest in life generally and enjoy the sessions more. They shared problems with each other and began to make arrangements to meet outside the group. Heather felt they were beginning to learn to support each other.

Specialised day hospitals and centres

9. Day hospital for older adults

This was one of a regular series of sessions for older adults attending the day hospital mainly because of their depression and loneliness, or to give relatives a 'breathing space'. Karen, the art therapist, always started the session by asking people to say their names, as they did not know each other very well and also tended to forget the names from week to week. She then allowed time for some introductory discussion, which often revolved around their ailments and tiredness, with questions about medication and so on. Many of them had considerable problems to cope with, so she felt it was best to allow time for a few moans before asking them to move on to doing artwork. Karen felt the choice of theme should give them a chance to reflect on their lives and how they felt about them.

She liked to use a warm-up theme to get them going gently. This time she asked them to write their initials and then make a design out of them. After that, she introduced the main theme – their weddings. The resulting pictures and their stories were shared in the group. Here are three examples.

(a) Edna drew a cinema because that was where her husband had proposed to her. She had also drawn her trousseau, kitchen cloths and towels, eiderdowns – all very practical items. Drawing this picture made her feel sad, as she had lost her husband fairly recently and was still grieving; but it also reminded her of the good marriage she had enjoyed.
(b) Doris drew a church and her blue satin wedding dress. Her mother did not come to the wedding, and she wrote this down in story form. Her father had given her a grandfather clock as a wedding present, and she had recently given it to her great-grandson, to keep it in the family. Knowing she was helping to create a family tradition in this way gave her great satisfaction.
(c) Phyllis drew herself in her wedding dress, which she had made herself, and her five bridesmaids in apricot-coloured dresses. These were very much things to be proud of in those days, especially as her trousseau (which she had also drawn) only consisted of some sheets and a table-cloth, because she was an orphan. She smiled with pride as she shared her picture, and she also said how different things were now. This reminded her of the many changes she had seen and weathered in her lifetime.

All the members of the group enjoyed the session and some came out beaming. They had shared reminiscences of one of the most important events in their lives, and this had brought them closer to each other. It also helped them to remember other events and they began to look back over their lives with a greater sense of perspective. Karen hoped that, in time, this sense of perspective might help them to cope more equably with their present situations and problems.

10. Alcohol unit

The alcohol unit was a day hospital which provided a six-week programme of intensive daily sessions in group therapy, alcohol education, art therapy, discussion groups, social skills and individual counselling for people recovering from addiction to alcohol. Both supportive and confrontative methods were used to help break down the denial and defensiveness which are often characteristic of alcoholism.

Part of the programme was a choice of activity on a Wednesday afternoon, when clients could opt for woodwork, pottery or painting, to help them learn to develop new interests. The series described below was part of the painting option.

The unit art therapist, Paul, and a trainee art therapist on placement were both available. They decided this would be a good chance to develop a series together. They opted for a series designed to bring clients into interaction with each other through the actual work, as this would reinforce other work going on in the unit at that time. Below is the outline of the series, with two sessions, the first and the last, described in slightly more detail.

Masks of others

The aim of this session was to prepare people to talk to each other by starting with something familiar. In the social skills sessions at the unit, people often discussed their 'fronts', their façades which they had come to believe were really 'them'. They were often unaware of their own, but could more easily see other people's masks. So Paul asked the group of seven or eight clients if they would paint masks for each other.

There was great variety in the masks produced. Some people had made several masks to show different facets, or had shown a number of facets on one mask. Some had stuck to sunny and cheerful masks, showing the 'brave fronts' adopted by people in trouble. Others had extended this to include contrasted happy and sad faces, as used in medieval drama.

One man had made collage masks by sticking on 'media images' cut out of magazines. An external mask showed pictures of a car, house, wife and children, etc., to indicate a 'successful family man'. Meanwhile, an internal mask of his real self showed a huge cut-out bottle with a monster's face on it, showing the destruction behind the façade. This mask also included a small cut-out picture of a 'happy family' crossed out with thick black crayon.

When these were discussed in the group, what came out was that people could identify facets of others' personalities as a half-way step towards recognising their own traits.

Mask of self

Members of the group made one mask or several to represent aspects of themselves; not only the sides they presented to the world but also how they really felt.

Body outlines

This session started with a relaxation session to help people actually feel their bodies and where their lines of energy were. Then each person lay on a big sheet of paper while someone else drew round their outline. The outlines were stuck on the wall and people filled in their own in any way they wanted. One suggestion to help them get going was to express any energy lines they felt in different colours. This session went very well and everyone seemed to enjoy it.

Section of body image

Group members chose one particular section to explore and develop into a painting, e.g. one person painted a bird near her heart.

Group painting

The group on this occasion consisted of seven clients (four men and three women) and three staff, two of whom did not take part because they wanted to observe the interaction.

Everyone started with one colour crayon, which they could 'trade' with someone else later if they wished. One or two people started off very strongly, but later modified their approach as the paper started filling up and they felt they had 'made their mark'. This gave rise later to a discussion of the need for control, which was looked at in terms of alcoholism, where it is often a key issue. The finished painting covered every bit of space, as if the group could not bear the thought of any gaps. This was often true of the discussion groups at the unit too, when clients found periods of silence most difficult. The discussion also covered issues of personal space and how much people needed their own space to themselves.

Paul and the student felt that the series had been a success thus far. The practical work had indeed achieved a good deal of interaction and had been enjoyable for most people. It had also raised a lot of personal issues, which had been discussed in the group, and many of these had a direct bearing on characteristic attitudes in alcoholism.

11. Day centre for ex-offenders

This example is taken from my work at a day centre for ex-offenders and others with social and personal problems. Members of the centre came voluntarily and chose from a range of activities which included woodwork, community service projects, discussion groups, video role plays, literacy and numeracy tuition, and art – either on an individual basis or in the weekly 'art group'.

Members of the centre played an active role in choosing their activities as this developed their initiative and helped them to feel worthwhile people once more. Together with me and one other member of staff, they had chosen to work on a four-week series on interpersonal communication. The 'Metaphorical Portraits' theme was part of this series and they were happy to try it. There were nine in the group that day – two staff (including myself), a social work student on placement at the centre and six members (three women, three men), whose ages ranged between 17 and 32.

I outlined the idea. We would all try to draw portraits of the other group members, not as they looked but in shapes, colours and lines to suggest something about their personalities. I was a bit worried lest one or two group members found it too threatening, or others used it to 'get at' the more vulnerable ones. In particular, one of the women was very unpopular with other members generally, and knew it. She was also overweight and very self-conscious about it.

We took about 30 minutes to complete our drawings, using oil pastel crayons. I joined in as a member of the group. Then I suggested that we played a game with the resulting portraits. I held one of mine up and asked the group to guess who it was meant to be. When the group had guessed, I gave it to that person as a gift, and she/he in turn held up a portrait of someone else. We continued until each person had a pile of gifts of portraits drawn by the others.

There were some predictable ones, for example, I received a paintbrush and also a series of brown wavy lines (my hair), but there were also some surprises. My co-facilitator was startled to find that one member drew him as a black cloud, and was worried about him. On the other hand, the unpopular member received several messages such as flowers, which suggested that others could see past her difficulties and appreciate her inner sensitivity. Just as important was the hilarity and warmth of feeling engendered in the group, all of whom were used to being 'put down' most of the time. The session had been very revealing, but in a gentle way, so as not to be hurtful.

This theme, with several variations, is a particularly rich one in that it lends itself to many situations. It enables people to communicate how they see others in an indirect and playful way, and also to reflect on their part in choosing a particular metaphor.

12. Cancer help centre

The cancer help centre provided an opportunity for people with cancer to try several 'alternative' kinds of treatment. Most cancer patients there came from all parts of England and abroad for a one- or two-week residential stay, during which they tried out all the treatments on offer, such as the special diet, vitamin supplements, relaxation, meditation, bio-feedback, counselling and art therapy. Relatives of patients were also encouraged to stay and take part in the groups. There was only one timetabled art therapy group, so the art therapist, Heather, felt the session should open as many doors as possible for people which they could explore later on their own.

The cancer patients attending the centre were very much 'normal people' who had had the ground cut from under their feet by their illness. They found it difficult to have any concept of the future without feeling that they were looking into their own graves. Much of therapy has traditionally paid most of its attention to blockages in the past, but here was a setting where the blockage seemed to be in the future. Therefore Heather wanted to suggest a theme that might help them to look at the future again in a positive way.

In this particular session she took the group on an imaginary journey down under the sea, swimming through an underwater cave to come up at an island where they met someone who gave them a gift. She asked people to paint the gift and the person who gave it to them. The resulting pictures were fascinating. Several of the gifts were beautiful shells or shimmering jewels, which could be seen as gifts of life. In some of the pictures sharks hovered, preventing them from reaching the gifts. It was not difficult to relate the sharks to symbols of death or their cancer. In the discussion that followed, some of the group linked acceptance of these gifts with being able to anticipate the future once more.

On another occasion I was standing in for Heather, who was on holiday. There were five people in the group, all in their first week at the centre: David, a cancer patient in his thirties; Tom, a cancer patient in his fifties and his wife Sheila; Tanya and Jeanette, daughters of a cancer patient who was too tired to attend the session. After introductions all round and explaining the nature of the session, I introduced another 'journey' theme: 'A journey you would like to make, or one you have already made'. For anyone who did not want to do this, I suggested painting any image that had occurred in one of their meditation sessions, or trying out paint on wet paper to see what happened.

Most of the group really enjoyed the painting session and stayed a long while to discuss their pictures – and personal painting in general. Tanya and Jeanette had come to find out how to help their mother to start painting, as they felt this might help her to recover from cancer. They painted with enthusiasm, and we also discussed specific ideas for them to try with their mother when she felt ready. David had painted a meticulous picture of a journey to Cyprus, where he and his girlfriend were going on holiday later in the year (and had been before). He also painted a second picture – an abstract with much looser flowing lines – and was keen to continue exploring this way of painting when he returned home. He felt the cancer help centre had given him a new attitude and a new lease of life, and was determined to win through. He was a workaholic businessman and felt that painting and music might be very useful ways for him to relax on his own and discover his personal life once more. Only Tom did not enjoy the session. He had never painted and could not mix the colours he wanted, yet resisted my offers to help – as if he could not admit to ignorance. His painting consisted of a few unconnected blobs and bands and he did not finish it. Sheila had enjoyed doing her painting, but when Tom left early she followed suit.

At the end of the session, everyone helped to clear up and I felt happy that I had been able to suggest a possible direction to three of the group. I also felt very privileged to have witnessed the courage and determination of these people, who were trying to carve out a positive purpose in the face of death.

These two rather different sessions show some of the benefits of art therapy for cancer patients. It can open doors to personal communication about 'unspeakable' things, and help to resolve feelings connected with these – and the uncertain future which most cancer patients face.

13. Children experiencing difficulties

This was a group of nine 9-year-olds (eight boys and one girl), who were withdrawn from ordinary schools for one afternoon a week because they had family problems and were finding school difficult. The purpose of the afternoon was to give them extra attention and a chance to play. They spent an hour on artwork, then a short while on movement and trust games, after which came a break for juice and biscuits, followed by free play with a variety of toys, games and apparatus. The group had been attending these sessions for five weeks. They were a very active group of children and quite difficult to handle.

Heather's main method of working was to try to activate the children's imaginations and draw on their rich fantasy life. She usually started with some discussion, leading into a theme by making up stories that led them into imaginary situations that they could fit around themselves.

Family tree

In this session, Heather wanted to look at the children's family relationships in as wide a sense as possible, i.e. those people the children related to most strongly. She introduced the theme by talking about fairy-tale relatives, using Cinderella as an example to draw out the children's views on 'nice' and 'horrible' relatives. Then she asked the children to close their eyes and imagine they were going out to play one evening and climbed up a favourite tree with a tree-house in it, where they fell asleep. When they woke, they found it was morning and they could hear a dawn chorus. But when they looked out, instead of birds, they saw all sorts of their relatives calling to them, some climbing up the tree towards them, others perhaps falling out of the tree – and so on. After they had had a little time to imagine this, Heather asked them to open their eyes and paint their 'Family tree'.

The results were varied. One boy missed the point (or decided to do his own thing) and painted his new toy car. Most of the group enjoyed the possibility of people falling out of the tree, and made sure it was the 'unfavourite' relatives who did the falling. All kinds of people climbed in and out of their trees, and the people most important to them tended to be in evidence in prominent positions. The girl in the group painted a big round tree which (Heather noticed) seemed to be the same shape as the picture of her 'Nan' which she had drawn the previous week. Her 'Nan' seemed to be the mainstay of her family.

Some children always finished before others, and Heather asked them to do another picture of their own choice. At the end, all the children held up their pictures for the rest to see, and said a few words about them. Heather did not probe if they did not want to say anything, and the discussion was usually brief as they were fairly restless by then.

Silence

This session followed on the week after the last one and was just before Christmas. Heather had been thinking about the children's need to have a space for something to come up inside themselves and tried to link it to the Christmas star. Perhaps those who saw the star did so because they had been silent and able to listen and look? She asked the children to shut their eyes for a few moments and listen, to become aware of other senses than their most used visual one. They found this hard, but managed a few moments. Then Heather asked them to think of things that were really silent. One child mentioned stones. They reflected that even silent stones might help to make a noise when wind blew over them, rain pattered on them or water rushed over them. Heather asked them if they were ever really silent, and for most of them this was only in bed. She asked when others asked them to be silent, and it seemed that this happened mostly in school and when babies were sleeping.

Then they moved on to the painting. Heather asked them to paint silence all round the edge of the paper, and then to paint anything that came out of the silence in the middle. One boy painted white snowflakes in the middle. Most of the children painted themselves in bed at night in their bedrooms. One very agitated boy painted his father beating him up in his bed at night, which he seemed to accept as a normal event in his life. (This particular account was written before the development of many of the child protection protocols in place now. It is unlikely that professional staff would now let such a disclosure simply go by. To plan for such an eventuality, care is needed to let children know at the start of the group that confidentiality would exclude disclosure of abuse, and that staff would be obliged to act on it if disclosed. Then children have a choice whether they disclose abuse or not.)

After the sessions, Heather shared the pictures with other staff there, so that they could be aware of any special issues. The children enjoyed the art sessions and seemed to appreciate them for the personal space there just for them as individuals.

14. Asian women's group

The proposal for this group came from Awaz Utaoh, an organisation offering training, employment opportunities and social activities to women in the South Asian community. Staff there felt that art therapy would be helpful to explore and raise awareness of feelings and experiences previously hidden. They also hoped it could help members to look at current situations, particularly those involving anger and conflict, and possible ways of dealing with these. Staff suggested this focus because of the problems that members were bringing to them.

We held an initial meeting to discuss how the group should run and agreed that I would hold the group with my art therapy trainee and with translation help from the case worker at Awaz Utaoh. The group was to be a closed one, with six to ten women participating (selected with a view to their emotional needs), running for six sessions. It was held in the board-room – a quiet space with a large oval table, access to water in the passage outside and seating for 15 people. We brought two crates of art materials from our base at the inner city mental health service and drew up an information sheet for clients explaining the group in simple language. This included a programme of the sessions:

1   Introduction and ground rules – introducing selves on paper.
2   What is anger? How do we express it?
3   What is underneath anger? A look at some of the causes.
4   Family issues – how do they relate to anger?
5   Anger and empowerment – being assertive.
6   Review and plans for moving on.

In the event things worked out rather differently from the way Awaz Utaoh had envisaged. First, it became apparent that group members changed each time. For instance, the women attending session two were a completely different group from those attending session one, so we re-ran the introductory session for them. Then the course had to be shortened to five sessions as a Muslim festival clashed with one of the art therapy sessions. We also changed the starting time of the group from 11.00 to 11.30 as very few people had arrived by 11.00 am. So we ended up omitting sessions four and six on the list above.

Altogether 18 women attended, a mixture of middle-aged and young women (who left their children in the crèche and often had to leave the group to attend to them). No one attended all five sessions, but two women (both mental health clients about whom the centre was worried) attended four sessions. A few others attended three or two sessions and 13 women attended just one of the sessions. The attendance each week varied between four and nine women. My art therapy trainee (Helen), the case worker helping with translation (Nazlin) and I attended each week and also participated in the artwork. Nazlin's participation was especially helpful in enabling the women to make a start.

Session 1

A total of nine women attended, all coming in at different times. Most spoke some English but it was very useful to have Nazlin as interpreter. I explained the principles of art therapy to the group. These were received with much interest, humour and lively comment, enabling the facilitators to explore any worries or fears about the sessions. I went over the ground rules including confidentiality, the right to pass (i.e. not join in, if something felt difficult or uncomfortable), respect, punctuality and clearing up. The theme for the day was introducing themselves on paper in whatever way they wanted.

For the first session we used dry materials only: felt tip pens, pastels, crayons. The whole group participated, including the facilitators. After completing their pictures, members of the group were invited to talk about them. This produced much laughter and some sadness. Everyone chose to talk about their picture.

Session 2

This session was slow to start because, as Nazlin explained, many women had got back late from an Awaz Utaoh trip to Birmingham the previous day. An entirely different set of women finally assembled, so I decided to re-run the introductory session of the previous week and extend the session to 12.15 so that everyone would have a chance to draw or paint. Paints were introduced and proved very popular, resulting in some wonderfully self-introductory pictures. A very lively discussion arose about colour symbolism and a comparison between colour meanings in Indian and British culture. Black was a positive shade not associated with death. White was worn at Indian funerals. Red did not denote anger but was used a lot at weddings.

Session 3

This session started at the revised time of 11.30 am, which seemed more convenient for the group. Five women turned up, four of whom had attended other sessions. This enabled me to introduce the theme 'What is anger? How do we express it?' to the group. I asked what anger looked like in terms of shapes and colours. What sorts of things make us angry – people, family, situations? How are we affected by other people's anger?

Nazlin's skilful translation into several different languages and her understanding of art therapy conveyed the subtleties of the theme so well to the group that there ensued a lively discussion about anger in relation to their lives – sometimes heated, sometimes with much laughter – anger at children, in-laws, husbands, and so on. I reminded the group that they could ignore the theme if they preferred to do something different, but everyone seemed energised by the subject and proceeded to use the materials with zest.

During the sharing time everyone had plenty to say about the images which graphically reflected their earlier conversations. There were pictures of sons, in-laws, resentment at housework, continually clearing up dust, old kitchen units which needed replacing and an 'angry brain'.

Session 4

This session had a slow start but latecomers made the final number up to five – four had attended earlier sessions while the fifth was a young student who had only come to live in Bristol three months earlier. Helen outlined the theme: exploring the feelings underlying anger and how we often feel resentment about someone or some situation, but suppress it and then explode at some trivial upset.

Group members found it hard to get started, not knowing quite how to depict feelings, but I explained how to just start with making marks and the pictures began to emerge. Two of the group painted pictures depicting anger at husbands, one because her husband would not talk to her and never wanted to go out. The other showed an angry self-portrait shouting at her husband because he went to work and she got lonely at home. Two members showed angry feelings that had previously remained hidden, while one showed anger at a son who didn't perform a task he had been asked to do. The sharing time produced much discussion and everyone was eloquent about their pictures. Certainly a lot of angry feelings about families had emerged and been aired.

Session 5

At this last session four women attended, two who had attended three other sessions and two newcomers who had art therapy explained to them by Nazlin. In view of the shortened number of sessions, we had to miss out two of the planned topics, but we felt it was important to finish in a positive way and leave the women with a feeling of hope. The theme was: a time when they had got angry but had found a positive way out of the anger. I explained that at the end of the session we would make a list of all the positive outcomes, so that everyone would have more ideas on how to cope next time when overcome with anger. After a slow start, a growing sense of intense concentration resulted in some striking pictures, with free use of paint, felt-tip pens and crayons.

During the sharing time, group members described their pictures and their coping mechanisms, which I wrote up on large sheets of paper. One woman got angry with the weather, especially if it didn't rain, as in her country of origin no rain makes people anxious. What helped her was praying. Another member drew a picture of her daughter and explained that when she got angry with her daughter undeservedly, she then did nice things for her to make up for the anger (Figure 6.4).

Another member contributed terrible tales of racism and victimisation while running a shop. She dealt with it by leaving the shop to take over a petrol station. Her way of coping was to find people she liked to communicate with. The fourth member of the group drew a picture of the park she went to when angry with her husband, as she found the park calming.

At the end of the sharing time, the list contained 20 ways of coping with anger. Then followed an interesting discussion on the role of women in Asian culture – early marriage and children, usually involving 'marrying the husband's family' as most women move to live with their in-laws. Many of them wanted changes for their children. They were unanimous in their approval of girls as well as boys getting a good education and career first before thinking about marriage.

We evaluated the group by producing a simple form with four questions. Nazlin translated these for each woman who had attended (as far as possible) and then wrote down the responses in English for us to read. They showed that the women had really appreciated the opportunity to draw, paint and discuss issues which are often difficult to approach. The sessions were also notable for the colourful way the women engaged in painting, the laughter, the openness and generous sharing in discussion time.

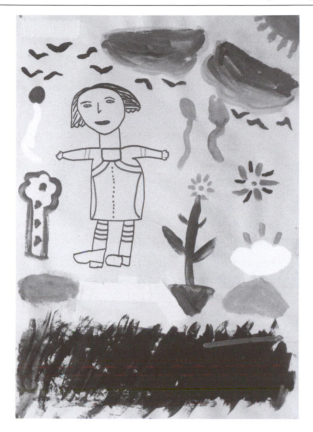

Figure 6.4   Nice things I do for my daughter – Asian women's group
Source: Photograph by Anna Coldham

Staff groups

15. Residential children's workers

Heather had been asked to run a one-and-a-half-hour art workshop for
residential workers in children's homes, as part of an in-service training
week run by the local social services department.

She decided that, as time was very short, the best thing was to start them
off painting. She pinned up a large sheet of newsprint on the wall, with
polythene sheeting beneath, and asked the group as they came in to paint a
joint picture in silence. There were eight people in the group. After ten
minutes she asked them to stand back and look at the picture so far, still in
silence. Then she asked people to continue for another ten minutes, trying
to work all the elements into a harmonious whole. When they had finished,

they discussed briefly how it had felt, both the painting itself and having to fit in with other people while doing it.

Next, Heather asked the group to do the 'Family Tree' theme, in the same way as she had asked the children to do it (see no. 13, this chapter). She explained that it was one which she had used with children and she thought it would be relevant for people working with children to experience it too. Most members of the group had related the 'Family Tree' to their families of origin and this had brought back many half-buried memories. It was quite a powerful experience for them and they realised the children in their care must also be experiencing similar strong feelings about their families. They were grateful for this awareness and felt they would have more understanding of the children in their charge as a result of their experience.

16. Staff at a day hospital for older adults

This was a group run by the art therapist for the six staff (all women) before starting sessions for the patients (see no. 9, this chapter). It aimed to explore the uses of art therapy so that the rest of the staff would be understanding and supportive of the art therapist in her work with clients.

Karen, the art therapist, started by explaining a bit about art therapy. She then suggested a warm-up theme: 'Make a circle, then draw something inside the circle and something outside it'. She chose something very concrete so that everyone would be able to do it easily. The different pictures showed quite clearly what people's preoccupations were. A nurse, who talked about TV most of the time, had turned her circle into the local television station logo. Someone who had just had her hair done drew a face with a hairstyle. Someone whose car was giving trouble drew a car wheel.

Karen used these to demonstrate how art can bring out things that are on people's minds. She then asked them to do a further warm-up, to get used to the oil pastel crayons. She asked them to do contrasts of light/dark, thin/thick, large/small, etc. Although some staff still felt quite strange about doing it, others were beginning to enjoy themselves. The main theme was related to their work:

(a) How I see myself professionally.
(b) How others see me professionally.

The results were interesting, particularly as they showed up difficulties between the staff.

Head occupational therapist

Her picture was the same on both sides, full of items of her 'practical occupational therapy self', such as knitting, kitchen assessment, home visits. She believed in sticking strictly to her role and showed no emotions to others at all.

Nurse in charge of unit

She drew herself behind a desk and higher than everyone else, and said how isolated and insecure she felt. She had only been there a year and was trying to get new things going, perhaps too quickly. The head occupational therapist had complained that she had 'overstepped the mark', so she had retreated behind her desk for the moment out of insecurity.

Nurse

She drew herself as being very emotional, but felt other staff saw her the wrong way because she said what she thought and felt. She also included practical 'nurse' things, such as injections and beds (even though it was a day hospital). In the discussion, the occupational therapy helper asked her where her soft heart was, which made the nurse realise that perhaps she did not show her soft qualities enough.

Nurse helper (1)

She drew herself in a waitress outfit, holding out a helping hand. She felt that other staff saw her as an 'Ever-ready battery' (which she drew) – always ready to be energetic and take things on. She felt she always had to accommodate herself to others, being grateful to find a job which fitted in with the needs of her children. She was relieved to find that other staff said they did not actually expect her to do everything, and gave her quite a bit of support.

Nurse helper (2)

She drew an outline of a hand with a large wedding ring; also a cup of coffee. She felt more confident at home and was not sure she was doing the right things at work. Others encouraged her that she was.

Occupational therapy helper

She grew quite upset as she saw what she was doing. On one side she drew a rectangle divided into small squares like a games board. In each square she put a different coloured circle with a black ring round it, with herself at the bottom. She felt everyone was 'doing her own thing' protected by their black rings. On the other side of her picture she drew yellow circles for her home life, which she said was much more sharing.

The session had obviously pointed up issues of hierarchy, role definitions, support, co-operation, etc. Some of them were surprised, and some felt it was a bad thing to bring these things into the open. Others disagreed and were grateful for the new awareness it had brought. Over the next few weeks, Karen noticed that they all seemed to contribute more equally in staff discussions and when they were working together.

17. Art therapy option on counselling skills course

This was a week's course on art therapy for adults studying for a certificate in counselling skills. The participants were all working in jobs involved with people: teachers, drug and alcohol counsellors, pastors, nurses, and so on. The aim of the course was educational rather than therapeutic, although the means of achieving this was experiential. The brevity of the course and the educational aim suggested that using themes would be helpful. I organised the course in five thematic days, with some reflection time at the end of each day. The numbers beside the themes refer to their descriptions in Part II.

Day 1: Getting into the art therapy process

- Introductions
- Squiggles (pairs)   no. 226
- Playing with paints   no. 35
- Introducing self on paper   no. 125
- Personal painting

This day was designed to help participants 'warm up' by interacting with each other in a non-threatening way (squiggles), relearning how to play and get used to paints (playing with paints), gel as a group (introducing self on paper) and begin to use the art therapy process (personal painting).

Day 2: Metaphors and interpretations

- Guided imagery (plant)   no. 330
- Metaphors in art therapy   no. 164
- Interpretations exercise   no. 288

This day introduced some art therapy approaches (guided imagery, metaphors) and helped participants to become aware of the dangers of uninformed attempts at interpretation (interpretations exercise).

Day 3: Groupwork

- Sharing space (pairs)   no. 224
- Sharing space (group)   no. 240
- Passing pictures (group)   no. 296
- Group project: building a community (group)   no. 260

This day provided different ways of working interactively.

Day 4: Personal work, theory and tutorials

- Self boxes   no. 128
- Tutorials
- Slides of clients' art therapy work
- Theory and discussion

This morning and the next provided the time and space for participants to engage in a longer personal piece of work (self boxes). Alongside this they had individual tutorials to discuss their assignments. The afternoon, which was given over to slides of client work, gave a glimpse of how art therapy worked in practice.

Day 5: Personal work, tutorials and closing

- Self boxes (continued)
- Tutorials
- Group gifts   no. 282
- Evaluation forms

The morning continued the personal space and tutorials and the afternoon provided a group ritual closing of the course. It would take too long to describe the whole week in detail, so I have chosen two exercises, a group project and an individual exercise, which are described below. Readers can build up a picture of the rest of the week by following up the exercises from their numbers.

Group project: Building a community (Day 3)

The group project 'Building a community' on Day 3 took most of the afternoon. We taped four sheets of card to several tables pushed together, and arranged the bag of clay and binliners full of 'junk' in a convenient position. Paints and crayons were also accessible. I asked the group to build

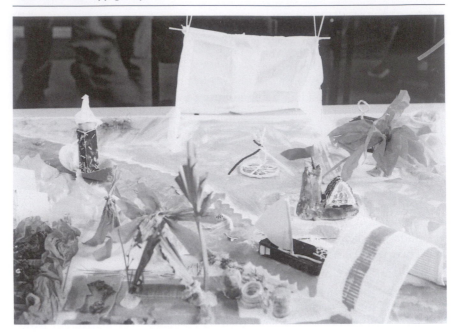

Figure 6.5   Building a community – counselling skills course
Source: Photograph by Sue Barrance

a community on the card, and to include whatever they thought might be needed. I also asked the group to work in silence as far as possible so that the communication would be through the media.

After a short pause of hesitation, everyone got busy with their own contribution. Some people worked away from the table and brought a finished object to place in the right position, such as the church placed in the centre by the river, the two boats and the fire (see Figure 6.5). Others worked directly on the card, to make a garden (see foreground) or paint the river. Several palm trees were added, a house and bananas and other fruits. As more things appeared, people began to work together, adding things to each other's work or holding things down while the other person taped or stuck them to the card. Two people worked together to complete a large tent which they taped to the edge of the card. One person spent a long time quietly modelling a food and cooking area (see Figure 6.6), 'lost in her own child's world' as she put it. Another person used brownish-yellow paint to unify the whole community – and suddenly it seemed finished.

As a way of processing the experience, I asked the group to write for a few minutes about the experience, or the end result and what it meant to them – a poem, prose or just a list of words. One participant contributed a poem:

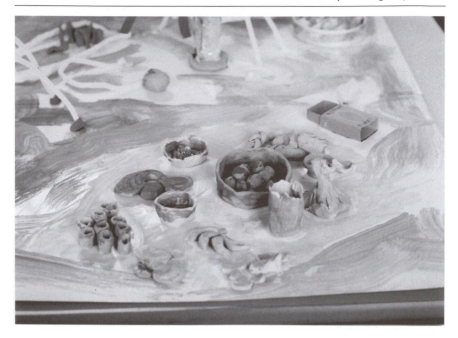

Figure 6.6   Building a community: the cooking corner − counselling skills course
Source: Photograph by Sue Barrance

As I was sitting on the Island
Something occurred today
That I need other people
To maybe come and play

The first thing that came to mind
Was the shading of the trees
And the bananas there within the leaves
Swaying in the breeze

Next thing that came to me
A house right by the sea
With big wide doors and decking
And room for me to be

Alone if I so chose it
With company close by
[and then all the members of the group are listed]

The general consensus was that they had indeed built a community where
they would like to live. All the vital services were there − food, shelter, fire,

water, fish, bananas, even some hammocks. Survival and working together were key aspects, but the element of play also stood out. For several people this had been something missing from their childhood, and most of them currently had fairly pressured lives, with full- or part-time jobs, families and the counselling course commitments on top of these.

This exercise does not always work out harmoniously, and sometimes there is a lot to learn from the conflicts that arise. One participant wondered if this group would have learnt more if there had been more conflict. Often people unconsciously take up roles they occupy in other groups (e.g. the initiator, the background worker, the finisher, etc.), and this exercise provides an opportunity to reflect on these roles. The important thing is to be flexible and work with whichever aspect arises for a particular group.

Self boxes (Days 4 and 5)

This was a very personal exercise, which can only be done with a group that has built up some trust. It fitted into the course well towards the end of the week, when I had to make time for individual tutorials for everyone in the group. I introduced the exercise by explaining that we could think of ourselves as having a public self, which we showed to others, and an inner self, which we only showed to some people or to no one. I provided a pile of cardboard boxes of different shapes and sizes, and the whole range of art materials was available as usual. There would be many ways of interpreting this exercise, as each person made it their own. I encouraged people not to work it all out beforehand, but to start with their first idea and let one idea lead to another in an organic way.

We shared the resulting boxes at the end of the morning on the last day. It was a very moving session, as people shared some very personal things, sometimes for the first time. Having the boxes there in the concrete reality facilitated this. However, I was careful to emphasise that there should be no pressure to 'reveal all' and some people kept certain parts literally 'under wraps' while being quite happy to share other aspects. The variety was breathtaking: boxes within boxes; collage from magazines outside and inside; use of junk materials to create textures with personal meanings; clay and plasticine models of little people; constructions with several levels, and more. As well as being an opportunity to explore aspects of the self, the sharing was also an occasion to celebrate the variety of interpretations of the same theme, and the creativity in doing so.

One person had an unusual interpretation of the self box theme. She disliked the idea that people might have completely separate inner and outer lives and produced a 'box' that was entirely open to view (see Figure 6.7). The different segments represent the way her life became divided up,

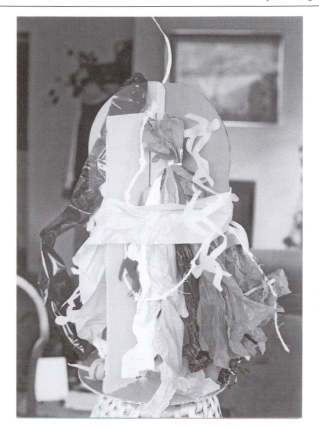

Figure 6.7   Self box – counselling skills course
Source: Photograph by Sue Barrance

but the divisions remain part of the whole. The full range of emotions was represented by the different colours of the segments. The tissue paper people were a reminder of the people in her life, past and present, linked together yet vulnerable. The shiny cellophane represented water and the light glinting off it, the bunches of tissue paper the interweaving of her life, with the knotted string linking things up and suggesting continuity. In another section she put an apple tree (poking out on the right) to symbolise the whole of creation and its interrelationships. Finally she added a pair of plasticine hands reaching out and communicating.

These two exercises both show how three-dimensional work provides opportunities for expression not afforded by two-dimensional pictures. Moreover the process of construction can offer extra insights. However, 3-D work appeals to some people more than others, as indeed the different contributions showed.

18. Teachers of peace education

This was a workshop requested by a group of mainly art teachers thinking about how they could promote peace through their classroom activities. It took place in a teachers' centre on a Saturday and had been advertised in the peace network as 'Peace Through Art'.

After some difficulty in finding the right room, most of the group arrived. There were seven people, all connected with teaching in some way, and myself. The teachers' centre warden, Steve, had been an art teacher and was very enthusiastic. There was one other art teacher and two former lecturers now running their own workshops. Then there was a teacher of children with physical disabilities, and two teachers of French, one of whom was about to be responsible for personal and social development courses at his school. We were three men and five women. I had never met any of the group before, but some of them knew each other quite well.

I introduced the session by explaining that we were going to use art as a means of communication, and that as art teachers they might find this difficult, or even offensive, if they had been used to thinking of art as an 'aesthetic product'. To relate it to peace education, we would try to look at the 'process' of peace through some interactive work, and see what feelings might arise. We would include work as individuals, pairs and as a group. We used oil pastels as there was no sink in the room or nearby.

Introduction pictures

I asked everyone to draw a picture to introduce themselves, their likes, concerns, lifestyle, anything that came to mind. As the group was fairly small, we decided to share them in the whole group. They were very varied: families, interests in sport, living on an organic smallholding, concerns about peace and the nuclear threat, French flags, etc. All except one (who turned out to have come expecting a lecture on the use of pictures) said they enjoyed pictorial introductions far more than verbal ones, and thought they could say far more in pictures. Looking at their own pictures, they also felt they had learned things about themselves. They thought this method of introduction could also be useful for the children they taught.

Conversation in pairs

I asked people to choose a colour to express an aspect of themselves, then silently to pair up with somebody with a different colour and have a silent conversation with that person on a sheet of paper between them. They could continue their own line throughout, or make one continuous line between them until their conversation finished. The conversations were varied: polite and evasive, friendly and harmonious, lively, or disconnected.

We shared the results in our pairs, and then discussed the exercise in the group. Most people had found the process fascinating, and also found it interesting to compare the experience with a verbal conversation.

Group painting

We taped together sheets of paper to form a large space and group members placed themselves around it. As they had come together as a peace group, I asked them to develop their own view of peace (concrete, symbolic or abstract) in their own space, then move out to meet others, resolving any conflicts using crayons (in silence). Thus I hoped to include the peace issue, both in the content and the process.

The result was most interesting. The picture as a whole was very rich and harmonious. People had worked well together and been able to resolve any 'boundary' problems without difficulty. The content, however, was another matter. Over half the group members, when they thought about peace, could not think of it except in contrast to war. So the painting included an explosion, a mushroom cloud, a bomber plane, guns and a black CND symbol inside a screaming head. This made people a bit despondent and we talked about the 'boringness' of peace as a major stumbling block to its achievement.

In our general discussion, the teachers said how helpful they thought co-operative work would be in a school system which encouraged individual work and competition between pupils. Co-operative work in itself would be a step on the road to peace, but was very difficult to organise because of the way schools and classes were arranged. The group thought they might make a start by doing some more workshops among themselves. In that way they could better prepare themselves to introduce the ideas and ways of working eventually into their schools.

19. Workshop for mediators on 'Art and Conflict'

This workshop was one of many to choose from at a mediation conference. Its aims were to provide a non-verbal medium (art materials) to explore aspects of conflict and an opportunity for participants to gain insights into personal aspects of conflict. No artistic skills were needed, just the willingness to have a go.

Several participants came to look at non-verbal aspects of conflict and to understand conflict in a different kind of way. Others came out of curiosity, to see how art could have a contribution to their work. Some came to sample 'something different' from the other workshops on offer, or to 'get away from words'.

After a round of introductions and stating some simple ground rules (confidentiality, respect, choose own level of participation, etc.), we did two exercises: sharing space and visual mediation.

Sharing space

This exercise is very simple but has profound implications. I asked participants to work in pairs, with a set of crayons and one sheet of paper between them. Their task was to share the paper in any way they wanted, without talking verbally.

Many different patterns emerged. Some pairs had drawn boundaries for themselves and then kept to those, working side by side but not interacting directly, although one or two echoed the colours and shapes of their partner. Several people said they had started by drawing boundaries or recognising 'separate territories', then gradually risked a small mark in the other's patch. Some of these remained separate images with small contributions, while others developed into joint stories in which the separate contributions were indistinguishable. One or two pairs experienced misunderstandings from their marks (as indeed happens in many territorial disputes) and became frustrated. The discussion focused on the variety of what had happened and the applications to their understanding of neighbour and other disputes.

One of the shared pictures is shown in Figure 6.8. This what one of the partners wrote:

> I have very little confidence in my artistic ability, but this didn't matter at all. A safe space was created where I didn't mind what the pictures looked like. I think this environment was critical for the exercise to work.
>
> 'Sharing the space' was a valuable exercise for me. It was like a visual tape-recording of my conversation, so that I could then reflect on it from a distance and see things about myself and how I interact with people.
>
> After a period of waiting for my partner to go first, I got frustrated and decided to start. I began by drawing bold lines and shapes across the page. When I noticed that my partner wasn't joining in, I became concerned that I was dominating and withdrew to the corner of the page closest to me, minding my own business as my partner began to draw. After some time, I wanted to communicate with my partner, but not in the same dominating way as before. So I began copying her drawings but with a slight variation – she had drawn flowers, so I drew a tree to keep to the theme. Then I drew identical shapes to her arrows but in a different colour.

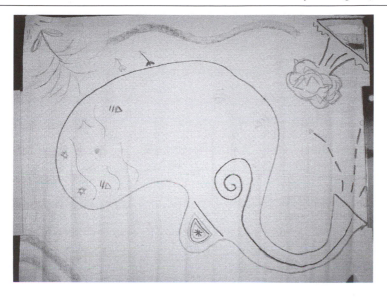

Figure 6.8   Sharing space – workshop for mediators
Source: Photograph by Madeleine Lyons

This exercise was satisfying because anything my partner added was a real contribution. This was a new perspective for me to take on in my interactions with people. Another thing I liked was the insight that conversations are always building something (for example, a relationship), in the same way that we were building an artwork. Although I contributed more than my partner to the page, and felt uncomfortable that I had dominated, maybe with art a neat 50/50 division is impossible!

(Lyons 2002)

Visual mediation

This was an exercise to develop a way of working interactively with images of conflict. I asked people to draw a conflict they were experiencing, preferably one which had two distinct sides to it – it could be an external or internal conflict – and then share it with a partner (a different person from the one they shared with in the first exercise). Then I asked them to do a new picture for their partner, using some of the same shapes and colours as their partner, but arranged in a new way. (This parallels the mediation process, in which a mediator helps people in conflict to see things in a new way.) Finally the partners shared the new pictures. After this we shared experiences in the whole group. Here is one participant's account of a work situation:

The first picture [see Figure 6.9a] is a representation of a situation with which I am currently involved (2002) in a professional capacity – an issue concerning young people and anti-social behaviour.

On the left of the picture I have shown a group of adults (dark blue) sitting around a table, drinking cups of tea and talking, surrounded by angry red scribble. The heated conversation leads them to affirm their perceptions of young people as a threat and the source of trouble on the estate. On the right of the picture, I have depicted the young people (orange), some racing around together, some apart from the main group. One individual is gazing in the direction of the adults, another is very small, lost and lonely. Between adults and young people there is a barrier (green) that keeps them apart.

The second picture [see Figure 6.9b] shows how my partner redrew the scene. We had little time to explain to the other what the pictures showed, so the redrawing and my interpretation of it relies on the whole on the visual material.

The scene looks quite different. Gone is the angry red, the barrier has moved and opened to reveal a lens. Now there is a means of each side having a view of how things are for the other. Each side contains blue and orange figures. The adults have moved away from their table and each is interacting with one of the young people. Adults have come into the young people's space and are interacting with a group of them as equals.

Interestingly, this is what I am trying to achieve – to find means of building bridges between the adults and the young people, and to enable each side to appreciate the other's perspective.

(McDonnell 2002)

Several people depicted family conflicts. Here is an account of one of these:

The first picture I did is about a conflict at home. It is about the state of my son's bedroom, a continual bone of contention between us. The picture shows the house and garden, with a lawn that needs cutting – that is one of my failings. I have drawn my bedroom in white and beige, a tranquil refuge [Figure 6.10a, right]. But I drew my son's bedroom in vivid colours to show my feelings – yellow, black and red [Figure 6.10a, left]. Actually I didn't notice the red (I normally never use or have red around as I hate the colour) until my partner redrew my picture [Figure 6.10b] including a large splash of red. It was then that I realised how angry I was about it all.

When I got home I showed my picture to my son, and he was quite amazed. He recognised my anger and said, 'I think I might have to do something about it – I didn't realise how upset you were.' And then I

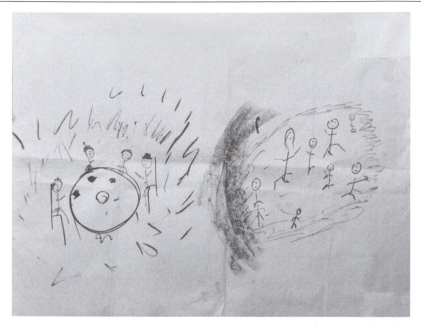

Figure 6.9a   Work conflict – workshop for mediators
Source: Photograph by Anna Coldham

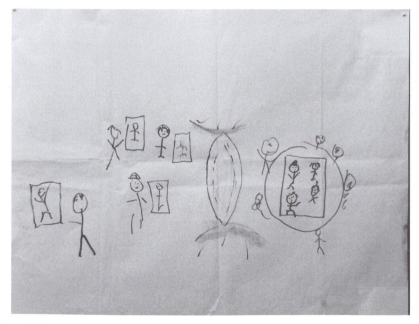

Figure 6.9b   Work conflict: visual mediation
Source: Photograph by Anna Coldham

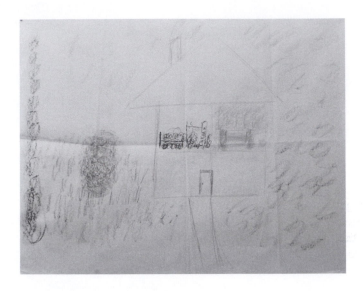

Figure 6.10a   Family conflict – workshop for mediators
Source: Photograph by Anna Coldham

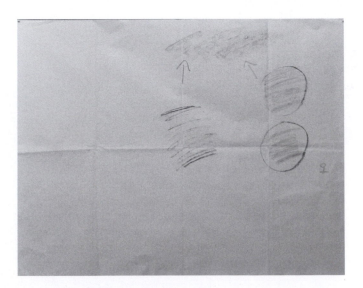

Figure 6.10b   Family conflict: visual mediation
Source: Photograph by Anna Coldham

realised that I might have unrealistic expectations of him, because he was always quite finicky when he was younger. It's been quite a journey of awareness through the pictures.

(Byres 2002)

Others portrayed internal conflicts, such as the following example:

The picture I drew [see Figure 6.11a] represented the internal conflict I experience when it comes to relationships. It revolves around a heart representing love, with a jagged line through the middle to show the two sides in conflict. On one hand I need freedom and passion in my life – this is represented by the left-hand side of the picture. The blue sky on the left and the birds represent the freedom, and the red and orange in the left half of the heart represent the warmth and passion.

However, I also want security and commitment from a man, but this doesn't seem to be harmonious with the other needs. So on the right-hand side, the black represents the negativity and not being able to get what I want. The red tears represent loving a man who can't give me the security and love that I want. The ball and chain represent being trapped by men that are interested in me but who are not interesting to me.

The picture drawn by my workshop partner [Figure 6.11b] puts a different perspective on my perceived conflict. She has taken the heart and put roots underneath it for the security I want, and above it bluebirds for freedom. In doing this, she shows that security and freedom can be in harmony. She has put some red tears at the end of the birds to show that life does have tears but they do not dominate the picture, and in the same way, they do not dominate life. In the heart, she has used red and blue to represent both passion and peace, and merged them so that there is no divide. On the right of the picture she has drawn a shoot with a heart, to represent opportunity and positiveness for the future.

(Taylor 2002)

At the end, one participant shared some insights about the process:

This exercise was also an effective medium for receiving 'advice' through a simple interpretation of my situation, and I experienced it as a real contribution. I was more open to receiving this than when people tell me what they think I should do. It is quite touching for someone to take ten minutes to draw me a picture – it was a real gift, with no pressure on me to act on it, that remained my choice. I think the exercise worked partly because my partner was a neutral stranger, with

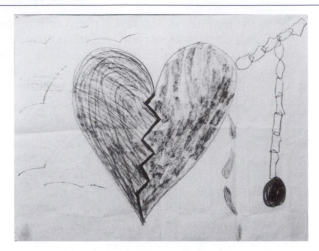

Figure 6.11a   Internal conflict – workshop for mediators
Source: Photograph by Anna Coldham

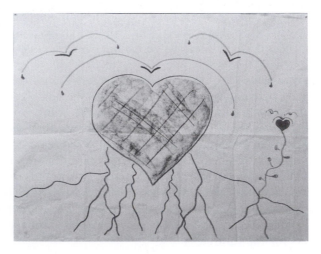

Figure 6.11b   Internal conflict: visual mediation
Source: Photograph by Anna Coldham

no ulterior motive, and partly because it was a novel and different approach. It has certainly stayed with me.

(Lyons 2002)

20. Race and culture workshops for art therapists

Two other examples describe workshops with particular cultural groups (see no. 14 Asian women's group and no. 23 Workshop for second generation

Jewish group). Many of the other examples describe a client group with a 'culture' of its own. This short section describes two approaches to issues which are often experienced as difficult. Using art materials can be a liberating experience in enabling conversations about these issues to take place in a non-threatening way. I have included them together because they were both workshops for art therapists grappling with these issues.

Workshop on racism

This was held at the request of a regional group of art therapists, who felt they needed to increase their understanding of racism and how to work better with race issues in their practice. I was a member of this group. The workshop facilitators talked about their own backgrounds and we introduced ours. They told us about their work and their experience of working with racism. Then they asked us all to draw an 'image of a racist'.

My image was of a punk with spiky hair, blue eyes, a Union Jack on his chest, tattoos on his arms, big leather boots and belt, knuckle-dusters on his hands, carrying a long thick stick, baring his teeth and shouting 'Go home!' at any strangers. I soon realised that this was just another stereotype, especially when other people shared their images. One art therapist had

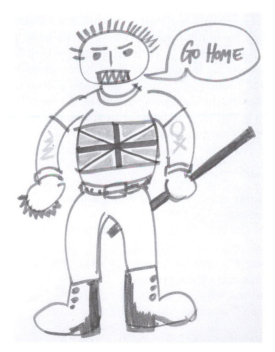

Figure 6.12   Stereotype of racist – race and culture workshop
Source: Picture by Marian Liebmann

drawn a white person among black people and said the first image that popped into her head was that 'all white people are racist'. Others talked about desperately trying to get the language right, but feeling confused about this and sometimes trying too hard. Several people brought up images from their childhood that had stayed with them.

This exercise led on to small group discussions in which we were asked to share stories about racism which had surfaced in our work, either our own or clients' racism. We were not short of stories, and this enabled us to compare notes and help each other with strategies for working more constructively with these issues.

Workshop on culture

This workshop took place at an AGM of the British Association of Art Therapists. The theme of the whole day was 'Taking Care of Ourselves' and the five workshop options in the afternoon all took this theme from different perspectives. The Art Therapy, Race and Culture Group (ARC) of BAAT was leading the workshop on culture. It was facilitated jointly by a black therapist and a white therapist. A huge group of art therapists opted for this (men and women, black and white), showing a growing interest in this field. A round of names and cultures showed us that we already contained within the group a wide range of cultural influences.

The art therapists facilitating the workshop asked us to do an image to show 'something in our culture or cultural identity which helps to nurture and sustain us', something which could be a 'safe haven' for us. It was a large group and the room was crowded, but soon everyone found a place and got to work. My picture was of a 'stream of life' in which tenacity and the ability to keep going were important in sustaining me. Because of the large numbers, we shared our images in small groups. Then we fed back ideas to the whole group for taking back to the next plenary session. These included:

- holding on to our culture without being a threat to others
- unity in the face of adversity
- relationship of the individual to their culture
- being sustained by others' cultures
- groups we choose to belong to, groups where we have no choice
- effects and meanings of migration
- what we resist and what we adopt of cultures
- the importance of place for some cultures.

We fed back to the plenary session the idea of a 'safe haven', a safe place inside ourselves which can draw on the many aspects of our cultures and sustain us through our work and other commitments.

These two vignettes show how issues of race and culture need not be 'difficult and prickly' areas to approach. The use of art materials can help to articulate the many positive and celebratory facets of these areas, and provide a basis for discussion of the issues arising. With the images to draw on, such a discussion can remain rooted in reality and take on board the many views that exist. Using art materials in this way can be an effective route into these issues for staff and client groups.

Community situations

21. 'Art as Communication' day workshop

This account shows some of the problems involved in organising events for the 'public', and how these can affect the experience of the day. It also demonstrates one way of constructing a suitable introductory programme, and how to include some flexibility. It is clearly impossible to include many details when there were several different options and a large number of people, so what follows is more of an outline.

This was a day arranged by request for members of the caring professions interested in finding out more about art therapy. It was advertised by newsletters, noticeboards and word of mouth. There were five of us organising it (John, Karen, Roy, Sheena and me), and we booked a church hall that was reasonably central and accessible. From the reply slips sent in, 12 people were expected and we arranged supplies of materials accordingly. On the actual day 23 people turned up. Several people had brought friends; others had assumed it would be all right to 'just turn up'. This posed several practical problems. Our small church hall was inadequate, but fortunately we could spill over unofficially into a larger (but cold) hall next door for the painting sessions, returning to our hall for discussion.

Obviously we could not do any significant sharing in a group of 23, so we divided into four smaller groups for most exercises, with one of the organisers in each group (the fifth one 'floated' to help sort out the many small practical problems). Even so, the small groups were too near each other during the discussions and found themselves seriously distracted by the other groups.

Other practical problems also manifested themselves: receiving money from several extra people took time; coffee had to be staggered to avoid long queues and waste of precious group time; we ran out of paper at lunchtime and had to obtain more. These unforeseen difficulties meant that the physical arrangements of the day assumed a much larger role than usual in determining people's experience. It was very difficult for anyone to get to know each other, not only because of the daunting number but also because the inadequate facilities did not allow for relaxing over coffee, for instance.

Nevertheless, everyone cheerfully made the best of it and joined in the programme as far as was physically possible. As facilitators, we took turns to introduce the different exercises in the programme, given below. One or two exercises are described in slightly greater detail.

Programme of the day

1   Introductions to the day and to the facilitators.
2   Name game: everyone in a large circle (rather squashed), throwing a bean bag to someone and calling out their name.
3   Introductory paintings: people introduced themselves on paper, then shared their pictures in small groups.
4   Coffee (staggered).
5   Conversation in crayon (see no. 18, this chapter for detail, and Figure 6.13). I found myself paired with John, and we had a slightly difficult time following each other round the paper. John felt he was trying to accommodate me and then felt trapped by this. I felt that I was having to take most of the initiative and got tired of the responsibility. We both realised that these were patterns we slipped into in our day-to-day lives.
6   'Round Robin' drawings. We started with something to symbolise ourselves, then passed our picture on to the next person to add something, and so on, until we got ours back again. One person in the group had drawn little anchors on several pictures. Although she said she was enjoying her present freedom and lack of plans, John wondered if her

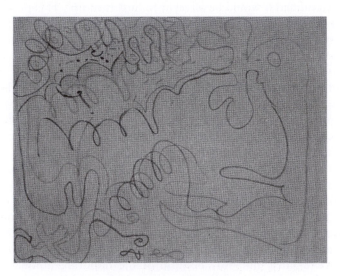

Figure 6.13   Conversation in crayon – 'Art as Communication' day workshop
Source: Photograph by David Newton

anchors showed that she was after all looking for a way of tying herself down. She looked at the pictures thoughtfully and said, 'Hmm, you could be right.'

7   Lunch. We put out everyone's food to be shared and people sat in small groups to eat it, or went for a breath of fresh air.

8   Choice of five different options:

- individual work
- collage
- colour exploration on wet paper
- group 'mandala'
- metaphorical portraits.

We had each prepared one option, but felt we could be flexible, so gave people a completely free choice. Almost everyone opted for one of the last three and we had to run two 'mandala' groups.

Group mandala

John was leading one of the two groups. On a huge piece of paper he drew a circle divided into slices, one for each person. He asked people to put whatever they wished in their space, including themselves if appropriate. It was up to them whether to demarcate their territory very definitely, to blend in with their neighbours, or to venture into others' territories.

Most people first used their space to do a personal picture. Although there were great contrasts, the completed picture seemed to have a wholeness about it. While two people chose to stick firmly to their own spaces, others were more adventurous and this resulted in more communication. Some were surprised at what they had learned about themselves: one woman, for instance, painted a grey volcano and then recognised how potentially explosive she actually felt. Another person found the negotiation of boundaries unexpectedly tension producing. For most people it was the first time they had attempted anything like this and they felt it had been a most interesting session.

Metaphorical portraits

I asked people to tear up a large sheet into eight small pieces and to draw 'metaphorical portraits' of each other; e.g. we might draw someone as a 'closed book', or just an abstract series of coloured lines. When we had finished, we played a guessing game with the portraits (see no. 11, in this chapter). As most of the group (with a few exceptions) did not know each other, we were rather hesitant and polite. Two people in the group received sets of consistent images – one of mostly blue-green self-contained shapes, the other of tall and closed in objects. At the end, one person said how perceptive some of the drawings had been, considering our slight knowledge of each other. Figure 6.14 shows the set of portraits I took home. Numbers 1, 2, 3 and 4 mostly refer to physical characteristics: my hair, height and the colour clothes I was wearing that day. Numbers 5, 6 and 7 refer to being seen as having a lot of energy: a revolving Catherine wheel, a waterfall, warm vibrations. The brick wall in no. 8 was done by the one person in the group whom I knew, and with whom I had had some difficulty in communication because of particular circumstances. She had experienced me as 'impenetrable', like a brick wall. Now, meeting at the workshop, she felt things were improving a little, as shown by the sun in the corner and the little green tree just poking out. My drawing of her, in turn, was a spiky, angular shape, which was how I had experienced her. It was useful to have these drawings to start talking to each other, and we were able to heal the rift between us.

All the groups came together for a few minutes at the end and we each said what the day had meant for us. Everyone was very tired, but also very positive about the day, and asked when the next one would be. Most people felt they had begun to explore themselves and others in a new way, and wanted to continue that process. Finally, we cleared up the paints, crayons and paper, wiped paint marks off the floor, etc. We were very grateful for a helpful and understanding caretaker.

22. Women's group

The women's group was an established group of 12 women who had been meeting every fortnight for about eight months. It had intended to be a women's peace group, but as many of the women were in the midst of difficult marriages or break-ups, considerable time was spent sharing these problems. Members of the group also saw personal exploration and consciousness raising as relevant to the long-term pursuit of peace. As there was wide experience within the group, we took it in turns to facilitate sessions on different ways of working. On this occasion it was my turn to introduce a painting evening.

I introduced the group by talking about the use of art for communication rather than to produce beautiful pictures. Any mark could be a valid contribution, and there was no obligation to join in. I suggested that we should try not to talk while we were drawing. I had brought with me paper and oil pastels, as the only room large enough for a painting evening happened also to be carpeted. We did three exercises: individual pictures, 'Round Robin' pictures, group picture.

1   *Individual pictures* on 'How I'm feeling', 'Where I'm at', to bring us into the present. We shared these in pairs and they were so productive that

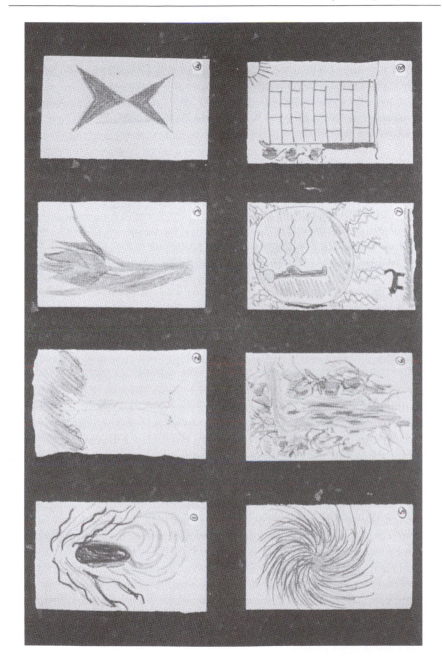

Figure 6.14   Metaphorical portraits – 'Art as Communication' day workshop
Source: Photograph by David Newton

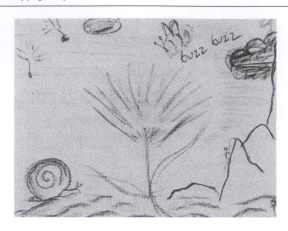

Figure 6.15 'Round Robin' drawing – women's group
Source: Photograph by David Newton

(with hindsight) we could well have spent longer on them. Fiona, for instance, drew an anguished red bird with one head looking down towards 'hungry beaks' (her children) and another head held up higher and looking beyond its cage (her marriage) towards freedom and the sun.

2   *'Round Robin' pictures.* We all numbered our papers with a different number, then spent two minutes drawing a quick picture. We then passed them on to the next person, who added something for one minute, and so on, until we got our own back. Finally, we had two minutes to put any finishing touches on our own. Figure 6.15 shows one of these. While most people in the group had been trying to add things that were in keeping with what was already there, Zoe felt we were all being 'too nice'. When it was her turn, she added something to shock the rest of us a bit, or give us something to think about. In this picture she put in the mountaineer scaling black mountains and the thick black clouds at the top.

   When we discussed our reactions to receiving back our own pictures, several people were thrilled at how they had been developed into interesting and beautiful pictures from their starting point. However, they were mostly quite upset at the black clouds and pointing fingers Zoe had put in. They experienced them as destructive and damaging. We spent a bit of time discussing how the same marks could be inter-preted in so many ways, and the possible misunderstandings that could arise from this.

3   *Group picture.* I suggested that we should 'make a base' for ourselves by drawing on the paper in front of us, then move out from our drawing

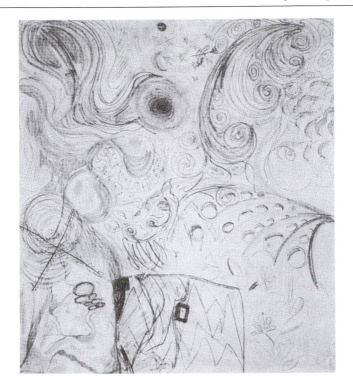

Figure 6.16   Group picture – women's group
Source: Photograph by David Newton

to meet others on the paper, trying to be sensitive to them (bearing in mind what had happened in the last exercise). The result is shown in Figure 6.16. The top of the picture looks fairly harmonious, with people finding ways of accommodating each other, even though some felt a little squashed. The bottom left, however, shows another story. Fairly soon after the start, Diana demarcated a large space in front of her in red crayon (bottom centre). Zoe and Wendy in the corner next to her tried to make contact with her by moving towards her boundary. Perhaps influenced by the previous exercise, Diana interpreted these advances as aggression, and first strengthened her boundary (top left corner of rectangle) and then withdrew to a small 'inner sanctum' (middle of rectangle). Finally, when they persisted, Diana reached out in exasperation and marked a large black cross on one of their patches. Fiona, further up the paper, tried to 'soften the blow' by decorating the cross, but it was too late. The rest of the group looked on aghast at the conflict the painting had shown up. Several women were not sure how to react at all. Afterwards we discussed our misinterpretations and talked about boundaries and their effect on fear and aggression. Did a boundary show a delineated space or a claimed territory? The last word came from Zoe, who couldn't resist the pun: 'Yes, it's difficult to draw the line!'

The evening had been a thought-provoking one, leaving several of us feeling a bit raw. Later I learned that Zoe and Diana had met for lunch to share their differences, and had had a fruitful discussion. They felt the group painting had enabled them to do this. At a later date the group decided to use further art exercises to help with communication.

The main use of art for this group was to help the group communicate better by introducing a non-verbal means of communication. By using group interaction techniques, a conflict which had been simmering for some time came into the open and could then be dealt with.

23. Workshop for second generation Jewish group

This workshop was organised for a group of second generation Jewish people, that is people whose parents had been Holocaust victims or refugees and who felt affected by their parents' experiences. They met monthly for discussions and support in exploring these issues, and decided that it would be interesting to try using art materials on one occasion. The workshop took place on a Sunday all day and was attended by eight people (two men, six women) spanning an age group from about 35 to about 60. I was part of the group and its facilitator.

We started the day with introductions (there were always some new people and two people had come for the first time because it was an art workshop) and ground rules. Then we spent some time playing with the art materials, as it was a long time for many people since they had done anything similar. Most of the group plunged in fairly readily and enjoyed the opportunity to experiment with textures and especially with colour.

Next we introduced ourselves using art materials. Again people worked with enthusiasm, using all the materials. The results were very varied, from coloured energy to 3-D creations celebrating people in their lives, including work and backgrounds. Several countries of origin of parents made an appearance. People were happy to share their images and experiences with the whole group.

One person had included food in her picture. This gave rise to a big discussion about journeys. It transpired that several people in the group still made piles of sandwiches to take on journeys (while recognising that food is available almost everywhere these days), as a kind of security, just in case: 'We don't know what there's going to be on the way, or when we'll find anything.' They recognised this anxiety as transmitted from their parents, who had done the same all their lives, dating from their experiences as refugees. Some people in the group also thought quite often about what they would do in similar circumstances: 'What would I take?' or 'Where would I go?' or 'Where could I hide?' or 'Where's a good hiding place in this house?'

After a shared lunch with a huge spread of food (part of Jewish tradition but also important for a group whose background included such concerns about survival), the afternoon theme was to explore 'Being second generation – what does it mean for us?' using the art materials. Some people picked up themes from the morning, others started afresh.

One person (not the person who had included food in the morning session) who was an obsessive sandwich maker did a picture centring on a sandwich, with colours and textures radiating out from it. She said her idea was to try to give up the 'security of sandwiches' and trust a bit more that there would be food along the way.

Two or three people focused on several generations and the links between them, also houses and holidays connected with these. Two or three others did pictures around the idea of 'losing the plot' or 'trying to put things back together'. One of these was in the form of a jigsaw, which was hard to piece together from one side (her background) but easier to fit together from the other side, related to assimilation into English ways (she had a very English partner) and represented by a coherent picture.

One person had pursued the colour theme from his picture in the morning. He painted careful squares and colours with the brightest colours he could find. At first he'd liked the order, then as he continued he began to find the order oppressive and felt hemmed in by it. He made a second picture using the same colours but this time just painted over the paper without any boundaries. In the discussion afterwards he commented on Nazism as the most structured social system ever, and related how his father had always refused to queue, on principle. This theme also resonated with other people in the group.

The discussion of the pictures took a surprisingly short time. It seemed that all the energy had gone into their creation. Another member of the group arrived and it was clear that it was time for tea. Everyone had found the day rewarding and thought provoking, and went home laden with their artworks.

This group shows how art materials can provide another avenue for people to share cultural backgrounds, both the common factors and the more individual aspects. This process can also give rise to discussion of issues that have been brought to awareness by the art materials. It is important in such a workshop to create an atmosphere of trust and safety, for people to be able to share vulnerable aspects of themselves and their backgrounds. In this case the group had a long history of being together, which enhanced the feelings of mutual trust.

24. Mixed group of adults and children

A church group annual party, attended by about 50 people (age range 2 to 70-plus years) was the occasion for an art activity with an opportunity for playfulness and imagination. After tea, the adult leading the activity asked people to form seven groups, each group to contain some adults and some children. He gave each group a large envelope containing a big sheet of paper, some sticky paper squares, sticky shapes, sheets of tissue paper, drinking straws, paper hole strengtheners, coloured sellotape, etc. Each group was asked to use the materials to make something to do with transport. There were no scissors or knives.

This meant that the groups had to work co-operatively to produce something. It involved all the people in the group, some of whom were elderly and had to remain on chairs, and some of whom were young children who needed help from adults to participate. There was a busy hum of concentration for the next 20 minutes.

Some of the finished articles are shown in Figure 6.17: a ship, a steamroller, a helicopter and a three-dimensional hot air balloon. Everyone was very thrilled to see the imaginative results. The children especially appreciated being able to take part in an activity on an equal footing with adults. Some of the adults too enjoyed an activity they rarely had an opportunity to do, and welcomed the fact that it was a co-operative venture.

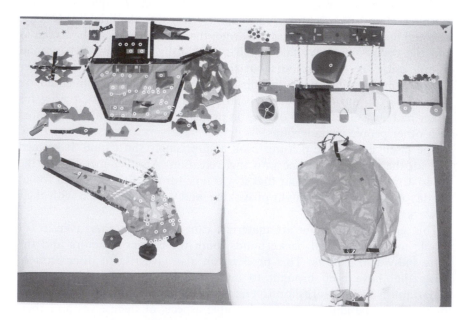

Figure 6.17   Transport collages – mixed group of adults and children
Source: Photograph by Heather Buddery

Although used here as a party game, this activity required participants to develop interaction skills such as co-operation and sensitivity to others in an imaginative way. These are all vital qualities in most life contexts.

Acknowledgements

I would like to thank the following art therapists for spending time with me, talking or writing about their work, for this chapter: Sheena Anderson (no. 1, admission ward in a large urban psychiatric hospital); Art Therapy, Race and Culture Group (no. 20, race and culture workshops for art therapists); Heather Buddery (no. 8, long-term community support group; no. 12, cancer help centre; no. 13, children experiencing difficulties; no. 15, residential children's workers); Paul Curtis (no. 10, alcohol unit); Karen Lee Drucker (no. 9, day hospital for older adults; no. 16, staff at a day hospital for older adults); John Ford (no. 6, day hospital 'Stuck' group); Marian Liebmann (no. 7, anger management art therapy group in a community mental health team; no. 11, day centre for ex-offenders; no. 14, Asian women's group; no. 17, art therapy option on counselling skills course; no. 18, teachers of peace education; no. 19, workshop for mediators on 'Art and Conflict'; no. 21, 'Art as Communication' day workshop; no. 22, women's group; no. 23, workshop for second generation Jewish group; no. 24, mixed group of adults and children); Nicky Linfield and her client Carly Dale (no. 4, young women with eating disorders); Linnea Lowes (no. 3, small therapeutic centre in the country); Richard Manners (no. 2, groupwork with clients with learning disabilities); Roy Thornton (no. 5, day hospital group looking at family emotions). I would also like to acknowledge the clients and members of all the groups described.

References

Byres, A. (2002) Personal communication.
Lyons, M. (2002) Personal communication
McDonnell, E. (2002) Personal communication.
Taylor, E. (2002) Personal communication.

Chapter 7

Starting points for specific client groups

The previous chapter gives several examples of the use of different themes with a selection of client groups. Chapter 2 includes a full discussion of the many ways of choosing a theme. It is worth going back to that section, to consider alongside this chapter, which includes notes on some starting points for specific client groups to help them engage with the process. These notes are not meant to be prescriptive; rather they are ideas to forward the process of thinking about your group. Every group is different and you will be the one who knows what will work best in your particular circumstances.

It is not the purpose of this book to provide detailed discussion of the needs of all possible client groups. You need to read about and attend courses on the characteristics and needs of your clients; there are many sources of information on these topics. There are now many art therapy books on work with specific client groups and these can be found through libraries and publishers.

The themes and exercises in Part II are not arranged in terms of client groups. Most themes are suitable for many groups, especially if they are used flexibly and adapted to meet particular needs.

This chapter consists of short notes on some specific client groups, related to their participation in personal art activities. Some client groups overlap, e.g. children and children with ADD or ADHD. Of course a particular client may be part of several different identified groups, e.g. physically disabled and suffering from depression. If a particular section of themes in Part II is suggested for a client group, this does not mean that other sections are unsuitable. It is up to the facilitator or therapist to look at the particular needs of the group. The letters of the suggested sections refer to the sections in Part II.

A note on terminology

In rewriting this section for the second edition, I became aware of how much the language we use has changed since the first edition. I have used the language that is current at the time of writing, but of course this may change again during the next few years.

Clients in institutions

1. Older adults in institutions

These are people who can no longer live in the community, and may be suffering from senility, confusion, wandering, incontinence, etc. For them, group art sessions will often concentrate on 'reality orientation' and activities which help them maintain their concentration on day-to-day tasks so that they remain able to cope with as many practicalities as they are able. For some, it may also be helpful to include activities which help them to remember their achievements, and give them a sense of dignity (see also Section 6, Older adults attending day facilities).

Suggested sections

- C. Concentration, Dexterity and Memory
- D. General Themes

2. Rehabilitation clients

These are often people who were admitted to hospital many years ago, for reasons for which no-one would be admitted today. Some of them may be in the process of rehabilitation to a state in which they may be able to live outside the hospital, with plenty of support. Others may not be able to achieve the skills of independent living and may never leave. They often enjoy art, but tend to repeat the same 'motif' many times, or can only engage in limited activities. Some will need very simple activities, but others will be capable of more, and activities to expand their skills and imagination can be relevant. These often work well if associated with a special event, such as a hospital or hostel trip.

Suggested sections

- B. Media Exploration
- C. Concentration, Dexterity and Memory
- D. General Themes

A few simpler ones from other sections, such as:

- E. Self-perceptions, e.g. no. 168 – Wishes
- H. Group Paintings, e.g. no. 264 – Contributions

3. Acute inpatients

This group includes patients with a vast variety of diagnoses and difficulties, such as depression, hysteria, psychosis, schizophrenia, anorexia, to name but a few. Often they will all find themselves in the same art therapy group, and the art therapist may not even know the official diagnosis of each patient. Generally speaking, any of the themes which are not too 'personally demanding' could be suitable. If there is a new group of inpatients, it can be useful to ask them to focus on the events which led up to their admission, e.g. 'How I came to be here'. It is worth remembering that some inpatients are not in hospital of their own choice and may be resistant to any suggested activities. Even if this is not a problem, many are in a fairly bad way and find it difficult to engage in a group.

Suggested sections

- B. Media Exploration
- E. Self-perceptions

Some chosen with care from:

- H. Group Paintings
- I. Group Interactive Exercises
- K. Links with other Arts

4. Inmates in prison

Prisoners comprise a broad range of people, with all kinds of abilities and disabilities. However, the security measures and surveillance in the atmosphere of a closed institution militate against any trust being built up. Most inmates survive the pressures of prison by protecting themselves within an outer 'shell'. Sometimes personal art or art therapy has to be done under the 'art' label, possibly in an educational class, and will have to overcome the image of 'chocolate-box' art prevalent in prison. There are a few prisons where art therapy is now practised in its own right. It can be difficult to establish therapeutic understanding in prisons, and it is worth remembering that security comes first. It is best to work in a supportive way and to avoid work on deep personal problems as this could be too stressful in a prison environment. Work with young offenders will need clear boundary rules.

However, from time to time there are experimental projects and pre-release courses which aim to broaden prisoners' awareness of problems and opportunities when they return to the outside world. Many of these courses aim to build up trust in the group and use a variety of structured groupwork techniques. Several of the themes in this book could be relevant, as well as ones specially devised for their situation.

Suggested sections

- B. Media Exploration
- D. General Themes
- E. Self-perceptions (adapted)

Pre-release courses might also try some of:

- I. Group Interactive Exercises

5. People in institutions: general comments

Large institutions often have a multiplicity of rules which, as well as being the only way to cope with large-scale organisational problems, are seen by staff as giving residents a sense of security. Personal artwork may conflict with this sort of ethos, especially if it emphasises individuality and exploration. Special care is also needed to ensure that different disciplines co-operate with each other and give the same 'message' to clients. However, art may open avenues for natural spontaneity and creativity, which can have many personal benefits. Care may be needed to find the best medium to use (e.g. wax crayons are easy to use, do not break and last a long time).

Suggested sections

- B. Media Exploration
- D. General Themes

Clients attending day facilities

6. Older adults attending day facilities

Older adults who are referred to day hospitals and centres for help often need more structure than at earlier times in their lives, as their problems (loneliness, bereavement, failing health, inability to cope with new developments, etc.) make them insecure. They naturally tire quickly, so that groups should if possible be held in the morning. Regard needs to be paid to the timetable, e.g. transport, mealtimes, etc. Attention is needed to accommodate all sorts of disabilities such as deafness, failing eyesight, arthritis, etc. Some of these can be overcome with thoughtful seating arrangements, magnifying glasses, good lighting, large brushes and crayons, pencil grips, etc. (see also Section 7 on Palliative care and Section 8 on People with physical disabilities, this chapter).

An art group can help older adults to reminisce and talk about their lives, the unhappy and the happy things that have happened to them, so that they can celebrate their achievements, see their lives in perspective and maintain a sense of dignity. The group can also celebrate current strengths and increase social interaction.

Suggested sections

- D. General Themes
- E. Self-perceptions, especially no. 148 – Life Review

A few of the following section:

- H. Group Paintings, e.g. no. 264 – Contributions

7. Palliative care: cancer patients and others with terminal illnesses

In present-day psychology we are used to looking for reasons in our past to explain present problems. However, patients with terminal illnesses face a blockage in the future, and this needs to be recognised. Themes which help them to face their uncertain future may be useful here.

Those who are terminally ill need an accepting attitude and an honest approach to the topic of death, which is often a taboo subject in our culture. They may be able to use art to express their feelings and come to terms with death.

Suggested sections

- D. General Themes
- J. Guided Imagery, Visualisations, Dreams and Meditations

Some themes in the following sections may also be suitable:

- E. Self-perceptions, e.g. nos. 140, 148, 149, 150, 155, 165, 167, 168, 170

8. People with physical disabilities

There are two aspects to consider here. The first is that of overcoming sheer practical difficulties, e.g. transport to the session, arranging wheelchairs, making suitable paint holders, using large brushes and crayons if appropriate. People in wheelchairs can even be enabled to take part in a group painting if brushes are tied to sticks and the paper is on the floor or the ground outside. Just arranging things so that a person with physical disabilities can use paint or clay may do wonders for their self-esteem and feeling of being a normal human being.

However, some people's physical disabilities prevent them from achieving the results they hope for and they can become very frustrated. Here it is important to try to use the physical disability itself to give a sense of achievement. For instance, an engineer who had suffered a stroke was using background washes and felt-tip pens to build up a picture, but was very upset when he could not achieve the straight lines he wanted and remembered from engineering drawings. The art therapist helped him to appreciate the new delicacy achieved by the fragile lines, and he went on to display his work at an exhibition of paintings by artists with disabilities.

Suggested sections

- B. Media Exploration
- D. General Themes

Some of the following:

- E. Self-perceptions
- H. Group Paintings

An organisation that may be able to help people with disabilities to paint is Conquest (see Resources section at end of book for address).

9. Blind people

Blind people can take part in art groups if special regard is paid to their needs. This means concentrating on tactile media such as clay, junk, textiles, etc. The Royal National Institute for the Blind (RNIB) is a useful resource.

Suggested sections

Please refer to the Media Notes (Section M in Part II) for themes which involve the use of collage, clay and other three-dimensional materials.

10. People with learning disabilities/difficulties

People with learning disabilities now mostly live in the community, often in small hostels or shared houses with some support, sometimes in their own bedsitters. Suitable activities can be those relating to themselves and the world around them; see also Children (Section 11, this chapter).

Suggested sections

- B. Media Exploration
- C. Concentration, Dexterity and Memory
- D. General Themes

Some simpler themes from other sections, such as:

- E. Self-perceptions, e.g. no. 168 – Wishes
- H. Group Paintings, e.g. no. 264 – Contributions
- K. Links with other Arts, e.g. no. 379 – Painting to Music

11. Children

Activities particularly suitable for children are those which provide starting points for their natural imagination and fantasy. This can also be related to the outside world and how they see it.

Suggested sections

- B. Media Exploration
- D. General Themes

Many themes in other sections are also suitable for children, and for some themes children's variations are listed. Some examples:

- C. Concentration, Dexterity and Memory, e.g. no. 88 – Map-making
- E. Self-perceptions, e.g. no. 129 – Life-size Self-portraits
- F. Family Relationships, e.g. no. 198 – Family Relations through Play
- G. Working in Pairs, e.g. no. 226 – Squiggles
- H. Group Paintings, e.g. no. 252 – Group Murals on Themes
- I. Group Interactive Exercises, e.g. no. 307 – Animal Consequences
- J. Guided Imagery, Visualisations, Dreams and Meditations, e.g. no. 317 – Magic Carpet Ride
- K. Links with other Arts, e.g. no. 359 – Action and Conflict Themes

12. Children with Attention Deficit Disorder (ADD) and Attention Deficit Hyperactivity Disorder (ADHD)

These children tend to be 'all over the place' and need help to focus and stick to one thing. Pair work can sometimes help with this. Sometimes children are worried and themes that help them to express their fears can be useful. Often they are confused and angry, and activities that help them vent anger harmlessly can be helpful, e.g. work with clay or other media that survive pressure. Metaphors and stories involving anger can be used to look at the anger. Within a safe space and some grounding, they may also be helped by themes that help them to get in touch with and look at themselves and feelings about family matters.

Suggested sections

- B. Media Exploration
- C. Concentration, Dexterity and Memory
- D. General Themes
- E. Self-perceptions, e.g. nos. 134, 136 and 137 (Masks, Names, Badges and Symbols)
- G. Working in Pairs

13. Adolescents

Adolescents are often painfully aware of themselves, and frequently lacking in confidence, despite occasional bravado. They need the opportunity to try out their ideas and opinions without feeling judged. Many adolescents find dramatic themes catch their interest and help them to find a form of release.

Suggested sections

- D. General Themes, especially nos. 115, 121, 123

Many themes from other sections will also be suitable, as for Children (Section 11, this chapter), and adolescents may be able to use a wider selection from some sections.

14. Children and adults with autistic spectrum disorders

Children and adults with this disorder include those with autism and Asperger's syndrome, covering a wide range of abilities, from those without speech to university graduates. What they have in common is an inability to understand other people's feelings and social interactions. This means that they need a very predictable environment and tend to get upset if things change. They often have obsessive interests and like to repeat themes in their artwork. They do not readily work in groups because groups can be unpredictable, so any groupwork needs to be approached with care, based on knowledge of individuals. Any themes used need to allow people to retain control over their world. Tactile and 3-D materials can be popular with this group.

Suggested sections

Carefully chosen themes (in conjunction with group members) from:

- B. Media Exploration
- C. Concentration, Dexterity and Memory
- D. General Themes

15. People with eating disorders

Eating disorders cover anorexia, bulimia and other less common eating disorders. Often sufferers are teenagers or young people (mostly young women, though not all) who are high achievers and 'perfectionists'. The most common disorder to be referred for treatment is anorexia because it can be life threatening. Some people go through phases of anorexia and then bulimia. Some therapists may find body image themes useful (although not all agree on this); others concentrate on the emotional turmoil that lies behind the disorder. Anorexia sufferers often need to start with materials they can control, later moving on to materials which are less controllable. Bulimia sufferers, on the other hand, often start with uncontrollable mess for which they need to gradually find boundaries. Behind both these disorders may lie histories of abuse.

Suggested sections

- B. Media Exploration
- D. General Themes

When ready, some of following sections:

- E. Self-perceptions
- F. Family Relationships

16. Family and couple therapy

Here family dynamics are important, as well as the needs of individual members. Thus, many of the personal themes will be relevant for the latter and pair and group activities for the former. For families with problems, art activities may also be a source of shared pleasure which may have been lacking for some time.

Suggested sections

FAMILY DYNAMICS

- F. Family Relationships
- G. Working in Pairs
- H. Group Paintings
- I. Group Interactive Exercises

INDIVIDUAL NEEDS

- E. Self-perceptions

If children are involved, see also themes for Children (Section 11, this chapter).

17. Clients with mental health problems

A wide variety of themes will be relevant here, depending on the nature of the group and the particular needs. They may include very different kinds of people, capable of different levels of insight, and the choice of theme will need to be varied accordingly. Day centre clients are often involved in outside activities and relationships. These can be used as material for art groups.

Suggested sections

All section can be used, bearing in mind the needs of each group and the individuals in it.

18. Probation clients and young offenders being supervised

Offenders include a vast range of people with different needs and abilities. Again, levels of insight will vary and the choice of theme or activity should be tailored to the group's needs. Groups may need firm boundary rules along with encouragement to engage. Often themes will need to reflect their offending behaviour.

Suggested sections

All sections can be used, bearing in mind the needs of each group and the individuals in it.

19. People with alcohol and drug problems

Most of the comments in the previous section apply. Many alcohol and drug treatment centres try to help people look at the pattern of events leading up to addictive behaviour, and at some of the issues associated with it. This often leads to helping people to develop personally.

Suggested sections

All sections can be used, bearing in mind the needs of the group and the individuals in it.

20. Workers in the caring professions

This group would include any members of caring professions, such as art therapists, teachers, doctors, social workers, youth leaders, church workers, counsellors. They can usually be assumed to have a fair degree of insight, but may not have used art materials before. Often they are particularly interested in the more deeply personal and group themes; it depends very much on the purpose of their session.

Suggested sections

All sections can be used (except C and D, which will probably not be relevant). Some may have a particular interest in Section E. Self-perceptions. It may be good to start with a warm-up from Section B. Media Exploration.

21. General public

This includes almost everyone. The only thing that can be said with any certainty is that the facilitator may have very little idea beforehand about any problems that members of the group may have. This means being fairly cautious in the choice of theme and avoiding very personal ones until the group is better known. It is one thing to uncover a big problem and quite another to deal with it. It is best to keep the level of activity fairly light. Themes that can be interpreted on many levels are useful here.

Suggested sections

All sections can be used, but avoid themes which are very personal.

22. Other special groups

There are many other special groups and subgroups not mentioned here, e.g. people suffering from agoraphobia, women's groups, men's groups, ethnic minority groups, protest groups, self-help groups of all kinds – the list could never be complete. The main thing is to work out what the needs of the group are and attempt to meet them.

PART II

Themes and exercises

Introduction

Apart from a few physical and verbal warm-up games, this collection includes only visual art based themes and exercises. This is not to say that visual art themes should be used in isolation. On the contrary, they work well alongside other expressive arts (e.g. music, drama, movement, dance, writing). Many groups use several means of expression in the same session or over a series of sessions. There is now a substantial literature in all the arts therapies.

Although some themes are more likely to release strong feelings, this does depend very much on an individual's particular state at the time. The same theme can be lighthearted fun for one person and touch on something quite painful for another. Again, at the right time and in the right setting, it can be therapeutic to look at painful issues. At the wrong time and place, or without adequate support, this can be experienced as a disaster.

Because of this variation of response, it is only possible to include with the themes very brief notes on any common difficulties. The task of choosing a suitable theme or exercise and adapting it flexibly rests with the facilitator or therapist, who knows the group and the setting and is aware of the atmosphere and issues on any particular occasion.

It is a good idea to re-read the section on Choosing a Theme in Chapter 2 before embarking on the actual process of making a choice. Therapists and facilitators working with particular client groups can also consult the notes in Chapter 7 on the suitability of themes for their group.

The themes that follow may be regarded in the same way as tools which can be used in many ways, constructively or destructively, clumsily or skilfully. Following this analogy, one needs to know before starting what tools can do, but expertise comes with the actual experience of using them.

Classification of themes and exercises

This collection is divided into theme-centred sections, each with a brief introduction. The first sections are concerned with warm-up activities, exploring media, simple activities and general themes (A to D). Then comes a focus on the person, followed by a move outwards through relationships in families, pairs and groups (E to I). Finally, the links outward to other modes of expression are explored briefly (J to K). The themes are numbered continuously for easy reference.

Unless otherwise mentioned, most themes can be used with any two-dimensional medium, although obviously the medium chosen will affect what happens. Many can be adapted for use with less frequently used media such as collage, clay, etc. A Media Cross-reference (Section L) picks out the themes that make particular mention of collage, clay, 3-D materials and masks. Section M provides some notes on different media and their possibilities. These sections are followed by a list of the contributors to this book. Finally, the Resources section is to be found at the end of the book.

The collection was compiled chiefly from interviews with 40 art therapists in 1979, towards an MA dissertation at Birmingham Polytechnic. Existing collections in books and articles were also consulted. These are listed in the Resources section. The collection was revised and additions made at the time of writing the material in the first half of the book. The whole collection has been revised for the second edition (2004) and about 70 new themes added, as well as many variations on existing themes.

A collection such as this can never be complete for each theme can be adapted, changed or added to so that it becomes a new one; nor does it prescribe what to do. Browsing through it may spark off an entirely different idea which is not included at all. It is up to everyone who uses this book to add their own ideas and develop this collection in whatever way they want.

Checklist of themes and exercises

A. WARM-UP ACTIVITIES

Physical/verbal activities

1. Name Games
2. Quick Autobiographies
3. Paired Shares
4. Rounds
5. Handshakes
6. Mime Introductions
7. Mill and Grab
8. Group and Regroup
9. Big Wind Blows
10. Touch Colours
11. Body Slaps
12. Back Slaps
13. Shoulder Massage
14. Backboard
15. Pass the Mask
16. Mirroring
17. Pushover
18. Tick
19. Trust Exercises
20. Back-to-back
21. Lap Circle
22. Tangle
23. Knots
24. Simon Says
25. Birthdays
26. Breathing
27. Dynamic Breathing
28. Movement Exercises

29. Limb Wiggles
30. Circle Dances
31. Preparation for Theme

Painting and drawing warm-ups

B. Media Exploration, nos. 32, 33, 34, 35, 36, 37, 41, 43, 48, 49, 50, 53, 54, 61
C. Concentration, Dexterity and Memory, nos. 92, 100, 102, 104
D. General Themes, nos. 107, 110, 111, 118
E. Self-perceptions, nos. 125, 130, 136, 138, 146, 164, 183
G. Working in Pairs, nos. 220, 221, 224, 225, 226, 227, 228, 237
H. Group Paintings, nos. 244, 251, 253
I. Group Interactive Exercises, nos. 274, 296, 298, 302, 304, 307, 311
K. Links with other Arts, nos. 354, 355, 370, 371, 377, 381

B. MEDIA EXPLORATION

32. Doodles
33. Drawing Completions
34. Scribbles
35. Paint Exploration
36. Animal Marks
37. Colour Exploration
38. Linked Ideas
39. Opposing Modes
40. From Chaos to Order
41. Contrasting Colours, Lines and Shapes
42. Shapes and Paint
43. Patterns
44. Using Mirrors
45. Choice of Media
46. Large-scale Work
47. Using Parts of the Body
48. Left Hand
49. Left and Right Hands
50. Eyes Closed
51. Straight Lines
52. Creativity Mobilisation Technique
53. Wet Paper Techniques
54. Ink Blots and Butterflies
55. Prints and Rubbings
56. Monoprints

57. Working from Observation
58. Five Senses
59. Clothes Line
60. Just Paper
61. Tissue Paper
62. Collage
63. Scratch the Surface
64. Wax-resist Pictures
65. Textures
66. Using Found Objects
67. Junk Sculptures
68. Nature and Beach Sculptures
69. Mixed Materials
70. Work with Clay
71. Sand Play
72. Letting Off Steam
73. Working with Tactile Materials
74. Papier-mâché
75. Playdough
76. Slime
77. Creative Play with Food
78. Other Techniques

C. CONCENTRATION, DEXTERITY AND MEMORY

79. Planning a Garden
80. Domestic Animals Mural
81. Shelves
82. Shops and Categories
83. Breakfast Table
84. Daily Details
85. Clothes
86. Houses
87. National Flags
88. Map-making
89. Imaginary Traffic System
90. Objects
91. Fruit, Flowers and Leaves
92. Environments
93. Flower Collages
94. Experiences
95. Four Seasons
96. Natural Objects

97. Windows
98. Templates
99. Stencils
100. Initials Design
101. Circle Patterns
102. Patchwork Pattern Quilt
103. Weaving Patterns
104. Faces
105. Cut-out Shapes
106. Gifts

D. GENERAL THEMES

107. Making and Decorating Folders
108. Four Elements Picture Series
109. Appreciating the Elements
110. House – Tree – Person
111. Free Painting
112. Discussion Topic
113. Festival Themes
114. Eggs and Wishes
115. Design Your Ideal Place
116. Seasons
117. Themes of Life
118. Choosing Pictures
119. Memories
120. Colour Associations
121. Subjects to Illustrate
122. Islands
123. Action and Conflict Themes
124. Personal Experiences

E. SELF-PERCEPTIONS

125. Introductions
126. Self-portraits: Realistic
127. Self-portraits: Images
128. Self-portraits: Using Boxes and Bags
129. Life-size Self-portraits
130. Hands and Feet
131. 3-D Self-portraits
132. Sexuality and Gender

133. Celebrating Diversity
134. Masks
135. Body Armour
136. Names
137. Badges and Symbols
138. Metaphorical Portraits
139. Advertisements
140. Lifeline
141. Snakes and Ladders
142. Past, Present and Future
143. Life Collage
144. Life Priorities Collage
145. Aspects of Self
146. Recent Events
147. Childhood Memories
148. Life Review
149. Life Stage Concerns
150. Losses
151. Luggage Labels
152. Secrets and Privacy
153. Public and Private Masks
154. Good and Bad
155. Positive Qualities
156. Ideal People
157. Conflicts
158. Anger
159. Problems
160. Trunks and Dustbins
161. Empathy with Disability
162. Emotions
163. Feelings and Feasibility
164. Present Mood
165. Externalising Emotions into Characters
166. Objects and Feelings
167. Survival Needs
168. Wishes
169. Fears
170. Spirituality
171. Pictorial Narratives
172. Likes and Dislikes
173. Friendship Series
174. Perceptions of Self and One Other
175. Shadow of Self
176. Anima/Animus

177. Introvert/Extrovert
178. Personal Space
179. Personal Landscape
180. Safe Place
181. Personal Progression
182. Time Progression
183. Personal Time
184. Before and After Masks
185. Mask Diary
186. Reviewing Artwork
187. Institutions

F. FAMILY RELATIONSHIPS

Perceptions of family

188. Family Portraits
189. Kinetic Family Drawings
190. Family Sculpture of Relationships
191. Family Trees
192. Inheritance
193. Family Comparisons
194. Childhood Memories
195. Re-enacting Parental Relationships
196. Family Themes
197. Bereavement Issues
198. Family Relationships through Play

Families in action

199. Realistic Family Portraits
200. Abstract Family or Marital Relationships
201. Couple Relationships
202. Emotional Portraits
203. Present Situation
204. Important Things
205. Shared Experience
206. Problems and Problem Solving
207. Imagined and Real
208. Anger
209. Parents and Children
210. Role Reversal
211. Family Circumstances

212. Grandparents' Influence
213. Family Sculpture in Action
214. Family Drawing or Painting
215. Sharing Resources
216. Adding to Pictures
217. Teams
218. Art Evaluation Session
219. Other Pair or Group Activities

G. WORKING IN PAIRS

220. Drawing and Painting in Pairs
221. Conversations
222. Pencil and Paper Friendliness
223. Painting with an Observer
224. Sharing Space
225. Joint Pictures
226. Squiggles
227. Introduction Interviews
228. Dialogue
229. Sequential Drawings
230. Portraits
231. First Impressions
232. Masks
233. Face Painting
234. Silhouettes
235. Relationships
236. Joint Project
237. Joint Control
238. Power Roles
239. Conflicts

H. GROUP PAINTINGS

240. Group Painting with Minimal Instructions
241. Co-operative Painting
242. A Cohesive Whole
243. Moving On
244. Picking Out Images
245. Own Territories
246. Group Mandala
247. Individual Starting Points

248. Group Stories
249. Fairy Story in Time Sequence
250. One-word-at-a-time Story
251. One-at-a-time Group Drawing
252. Group Murals on Themes
253. Wall Newspaper/Graffiti Wall
254. Graffiti Anger Wall
255. Combined Anger Symptoms
256. How We See Each Other
257. Paradox Wall
258. Solidarity
259. Celebrating Diversity
260. Building Islands and Worlds
261. Group Collage
262. Feelings Collage
263. Creating Change
264. Contributions
265. Moving Closer
266. Group Sculptures
267. Overlapping Group Transparency
268. Group Roles
269. Role Playing
270. Painting to Music
271. Individual Response to Group Painting

I. GROUP INTERACTIVE EXERCISES

272. Portraits
273. Portraits by Combined Effort
274. Group Hands
275. Badges and Totems
276. Empathy Hats
277. Understanding and Recognising Feelings
278. Different Points of View
279. Cultural Identities
280. Group Symbol
281. Masks
282. Gifts
283. Affirmation Posters
284. Bereavement Balloons
285. Shared Feelings
286. Metaphorical Portraits: Individuals
287. Metaphorical Portrait: Group

J. GUIDED IMAGERY, VISUALISATIONS, DREAMS AND MEDITATIONS

1. Guided imagery and visualisation

(a) Preparation for visualisations

(vii) Support
(viii) A first-person account

(b) Imaginative journeys

317. Magic Carpet Ride
318. Wise Person Guide
319. Gifts
320. Secret Garden and House
321. Secret Cave
322. Doorway
323. Mountain View
324. Farm
325. Magic Shop
326. Boat Journey
327. Shipwrecked on an Island
328. Hidden Seed
329. Five Senses

(c) Identifications

330. Plant
331. Natural Objects
332. Dialogues
333. Moving Objects
334. River
335. Mythical Character

(d) Other ways of stimulating imagery

336. Group Fantasy
337. Relaxation, Meditation and Painting
338. Listening to Music
339. Breathing in Light

(e) Visualising change

340. Personal Development
341. Saying Goodbye

(f) Further reading

2. Dreams, myths and fairy tales

342. Working with Dreams
343. Daydreams and Fantasies
344. Clay Monsters
345. Stories and Strip Cartoons
346. Myths
347. Fairy Tales

3. Painting as meditation

348. Meditative Drawing and Painting
349. Mandala Possibilities
350. Autogenic Training
351. Colour Meditations

K. LINKS WITH OTHER ARTS

Movement

352. Trust Walks
353. Emotions
354. Gesture Drawings
355. Acting Sensations
356. Dance

Drama

357. Sculpting Situations
358. Dialogues
359. Action and Conflict Themes
360. Elements and Conflict
361. Accidents
362. Pictures Come to Life
363. Masks
364. Hats
365. Drama Games
366. Puppet Theatre
367. Theatrical Costumes
368. Storytelling and Plays
369. Tape Recorder

Words and poetry

370. Words to Image
371. Story Consequences Explored
372. Poetry as Stimulus
373. Poetry as Response
374. Concrete Poetry
375. Journals

Sound and music

376. Sounds into Paint
377. Name Sounds
378. Moulding Sounds
379. Painting to Music
380. Life Chart to Music

Multi-media

381. Letters
382. Evocative Adjectives
383. Scents
384. Stimulus to Paint
385. Response to Paint
386. Sensory Awareness
387. Music and Movement
388. Series of Sessions
389. Multi-media Events

A Warm-up activities

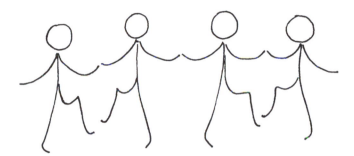

Many leaders and therapists like to start group sessions with some kind of warm-up to get people going. This can be a physical/verbal activity or a simple painting activity. The first will help people to get into contact with each other and the second will help them over the feelings of not knowing how to start to paint.

Physical warm-ups involving touching (e.g. back rubs) may not be appropriate for some groups: for example, where participants may have suffered abuse in the past; where participants have disabilities; where it is not an acceptable part of that group's culture; where a group is meeting for the first time. It is best to check with someone who knows the client group and what is acceptable.

Physical/verbal activities

The Resources section includes some books of co-operative games for those who want to develop these. Here are some examples, very briefly described.

1. Name Games

(a) Claps alternate with names round the circle until names are familiar.
(b) First person says name, next person both names, third person all three names, and so on.

(c) Throw a beanbag or other object from one person to another, saying name of person you are throwing to; or catcher calls out name of thrower.

2. Quick Autobiographies

In pairs tell your partner about yourself for two minutes (or five minutes) and swap. Then partner introduces you to another pair or to whole group.

3. Paired Shares

In pairs, each person has three minutes' uninterrupted time to talk about anything she/he likes. Other person listens with full attention.

4. Rounds

These are quick ways of sharing personal information and getting people started. Everyone in turn says a few words or a sentence beginning:

- On the way here I noticed . . .
- A good thing that happened this week was . . .
- Something I am excited about is . . .
- What I want from this group is . . .
- Right now I am feeling . . . (etc.).

5. Handshakes

Shake hands and introduce yourself to as many people as possible in the group.

6. Mime Introductions

People introduce themselves by each miming a characteristic activity or way of being.

7. Mill and Grab

Mill about, then leader calls 'Groups of three', and everyone gets into groups of three. Repeat for different size groups.

8. Group and Regroup

Facilitator calls different ways of grouping, e.g. all those with brown/blue eyes; all those wearing shoes with buckles/laces/neither, etc.

9. Big Wind Blows

Circle of chairs, one less than number of participants. One person stands in middle of circle, calls out quality shared by him/her and some others: e.g. all those wearing glasses; all those with a brother; all those who had breakfast, etc. These people change places. New person in middle continues. 'Hurricane' means everyone has to move.

10. Touch Colours

Leader calls 'Everyone touch red' and everyone touches something red on their own or others' clothes. Repeat for other colours and other qualities.

11. Body Slaps

Everyone slaps themselves all over, just hard enough to make themselves tingle.

12. Back Slaps

In a circle, everyone slaps the person in front's back (or all the way down). Then reverse circle and repeat with person on other side.

13. Shoulder Massage

In a circle, everyone massages the shoulders of the person in front. Then repeat with person on other side. This one follows on naturally from Back Slaps.

14. Backboard

People sit on floor in a circle, facing the next person's back. First person passes a short word on, by 'writing' it (with a finger) in capital letters on next person's back. When it has gone round circle, compare with original.

15. Pass the Mask

In a circle, first person pulls a face, then with their hands 'passes' the mask to the next person, who puts it on (imitates it), develops it into a new mask, which is then passed on.

16. Mirroring

In pairs, one person mirrors the other's actions. Swap roles and repeat.

17. Pushover

In pairs, starting in the middle of the room, each partner tries to push the other all the way to the wall.

18. Tick

In pairs, each person tries to touch partner in the small of the back, while partner tries to avoid this happening.

19. Trust Exercises

Rocking, lifting, blind walks, feeling and identifying faces, etc. (for groups where people already know each other to some extent).

20. Back-to-back

In pairs, sit back to back on the floor with knees bent. Link arms and try to stand up together.

21. Lap Circle

Needs at least a dozen people. Form a tight circle, all facing the same way, then everyone sits down on the lap behind at the same time.

22. Tangle

Hold hands in a line, then end person weaves under and round others until the whole group ends up in a tight tangle.

23. Knots

Stand in a circle with eyes closed, and each person clasps two other hands. Then open eyes, and without letting go of any hands, try to unravel the knot.

24. Simon Says

Facilitator issues instructions, which are only to be followed if prefaced by 'Simon says'. Anyone who gets it wrong is out.

25. Birthdays

In silence, using mime or gesture, get into a line in order of birthdays throughout the year.

26. Breathing

Sit with eyes closed, breathe deeply and rhythmically, drawing air right down, listening to breathing.

27. Dynamic Breathing

Keep repeating the sound 'who' while hopping from one leg to the other.

28. Movement Exercises

Simple movements such as shaking arms and legs, head rolls, stretching, awareness of limbs, relaxing, etc.

29. Limb Wiggles

Wiggle first one thumb, then the other, add fingers, arms, legs, bodies. Can also add moving round room and humming a tune, all at the same time!

30. Circle Dances

These are dances performed in one large circle. Choose those that have very simple movements. A music tape is needed and someone who knows the basic steps of a few circle dances.

31. Preparation for Theme

Physical movement connected with theme: e.g. arm-loosening exercises to introduce scribbles; spiral arm movements to introduce spiral lifeline; rhythm gestures to introduce movement to music followed by painting, etc.

Painting and drawing warm-ups

Several of the activities in Section B (Media Exploration) are good for helping people to make their first marks on paper in a non-threatening way. Some of the themes from Section E (Self-perceptions) also provide good starting points. Below are a few suggestions from these sections, together with one or two of the simpler ones from other sections.

B. Media Exploration

C. Concentration, Dexterity and Memory

D. General Themes

E. Self-perceptions

G. Working in Pairs

B   Media exploration

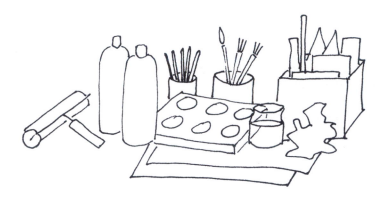

The ideas in this section concentrate on different ways of exploring media to develop imagination and creativity. Some of the suggestions overlap with or lead into themes listed in other sections. Many of them offer ways into using art materials and stimulate the playfulness needed to be spontaneous. They can be useful for new groups, or for people who are worried about making their first mark on a piece of paper.

32. Doodles

There are many ways of doodling, but the essence is to let a pen or crayon wander aimlessly, or 'go for a walk with a line', until something meaningful emerges. This is then worked on. Some variations include:

(a) Keep a 'doodle diary' and see if doodles change over a period of time.
(b) Close eyes to doodle, let the crayon draw as it wants. Open eyes, find image and develop.
(c) Use lines, colours and sounds without feeling there 'should' be an end product. Let a colour 'pick you'.
(d) From a number of doodles, select the ones liked best and least.

(e) Evolve a story from a spontaneous doodle.
(f) Verbalise feelings as doodle and something emerges.
(g) Squiggle in pairs – see no. 226.
(h) Metamorphosis: change picture in three moves to something else.
(i) Use dirty marks on paper as basis for associations to develop an image.
(j) Group can use marks on dirty wall as in (i).
(k) See also no. 54.
(l) Draw own initials as large as possible and use to find picture or design to develop. This can be less threatening than scribbles because the initials are already familiar.

33. Drawing Completions

From a given starting point of simple lines and shapes, complete a picture. The different results from different members of the group can provoke lively discussion. There can be visual (e.g. thickness of line) as well as symbolic differences. Variations:

(a) Start with a circle, make it represent something, then add something inside, outside or on the line.
(b) See also no. 54.

34. Scribbles

Use whole body to make scribbles with large movements, possibly with eyes closed. Looking from all sides, find forms that suggest a picture and develop it.

35. Paint Exploration

Explore how many ways you can apply paint – use brushes, sticks, rollers, sponges, textured objects, fingers. Explore thick and thin paint. Use different parts of the implements, such as the brush handle.

36. Animal Marks

Imagine that your paintbrush is an insect (e.g. a grasshopper) and make marks on the paper. Then imagine it is a snake and make marks as if it were sliding across the paper, and so on for other creatures.

37. Colour Exploration

Using one colour only and white paper, explore the meaning of this colour for you, e.g. by drawing shapes and lines in that colour. Variations:

(a) Select colour(s) most liked or disliked.
(b) Select two or three colours to represent a harmonious group, or express strands of personality, or show moods.
(c) Select colours to counterbalance negative moods.
(d) Start with one colour, then mix in another.
(e) Paint with two or three colours on large paper.
(f) Fill the paper with as many colours as possible as quickly as possible.
(g) Select a colour liked and a colour disliked, and make some kind of painting. Can go on to using two colours disliked.
(h) Do two paintings with colours most liked/disliked, and compare.
(i) See also no. 162 – Emotions.
(j) Starting with one colour, perhaps in connection with a theme (e.g. seasons), move to another, making a 'mosaic carpet' of colours. See if this gives rise to any particular image.
(k) Choose a large paintbrush and a colour, close your eyes and try to cover the paper with marks. Open your eyes and look. Then choose another colour.
(l) Coloured backgrounds: do a series of paintings on different coloured papers. Before starting, make associations with each colour of paper and use these to develop the paintings.

38. Linked Ideas

Work on a series of linked ideas or felt experiences by starting a new piece of work before the previous piece is finished. This can eliminate the fear of starting and promote a flow of ideas.

39. Opposing Modes

Begin painting in any way that comes naturally, then deliberately alter your approach and notice the effect. Repeat frequently while allowing notions of form to arise and be developed. Variation: Work quickly on a painting, then if there is a pattern, experiment with the opposite of what you usually do.

40. From Chaos to Order

Think of the word chaos and paint/draw in as chaotic a way as possible. Then stop and look at the result. Then pick a small part of it that you like and develop it into something meaningful on a new piece of paper.

41. Contrasting Colours, Lines and Shapes

Use colours, lines, shapes, curves, etc. to create contrasts: e.g. light and heavy strokes, long and short, light and dark, bright and dull, etc. Variations:

(a) Do just straight lines and curves, then reflect on which parts of your life relate to these.
(b) After working with contrasts separately, work on ways of bringing them together.

42. Shapes and Paint

Draw any shape you like, cut it out and add to it by drawing and painting. Repeat with a different shape. Variation: Stick shape on a background and add to it in the same way.

43. Patterns

Good ways of getting going. Some pattern suggestions:

(a) Repeated shapes. Choose three colours and a simple line form such as a rectangle, arc, etc. Use this shape in different ways, different colours, orientations, sizes, overlaps. If a pattern emerges, develop it with shading and connections.
(b) Repeat (a) using opposite kind of shape in opposite kind of way.
(c) Squares and circles, 'op art'.
(d) Draw ten bubbles and take line round bubbles. Fill in with colours.
(e) Take line for a walk – dashes, zigzags, bubbles.
(f) Make a simple shape and repeat it, changing a little each time. Form several of them into a pattern. Try using one colour first, then adding other colours.
(g) Tear out shapes and look at the patterns they can make. Then look at the spaces between the shapes and make a further pattern from these.
(h) Start with a thick wavy line, then draw thin lines on either side, altering the shape as you go. See if it suggests anything.
(i) Tissue paper patterns – see no. 61.
(j) Make 3-D patterns using paper, cardboard towel roll centres, matchboxes or other junk materials.
(k) Make textured patterns using collage materials or dabs of paint.
(l) Arrange cut-out shapes in a pattern, which can be altered from day to day.

44. Using Mirrors

Use wax crayons in three colours to do an abstract pattern in soft textures. Then look at the images formed by placing in corner of two mirrors at right-angles to each other. Variation: Group of four people produces pattern of soft textures, using one colour each, working in silence; use mirrors as above.

45. Choice of Media

Complete a given project in a single medium or mixed media. The project can be a set theme or left open. Reflect on the choices made.

46. Large-scale Work

Large-scale work using rollers, decorating brushes, sponges, rags, feet, hands, etc. Often best done outside in fine weather. Variations:

(a) Individual free expression on large sheet of paper.
(b) Roll liquid paint onto large card, then use shakers to shake on powder colour or glitter.
(c) Use variety of rolling objects to trail liquid paint from paint trays over long piece of paper.
(d) Group painting on large paper with sponges and trays of different colours around the paper. Group members move round every few minutes to sample each colour.
(e) Group painting with hands.

47. Using Parts of the Body

Use various parts of the body to paint, e.g. drawing round hands, finger painting, using palms and feet to make prints, etc. Variations:

(a) Use toes, heels, etc. to increase awareness of feet.
(b) See nos. 48 and 49.

48. Left Hand

Try painting with opposite hand from usual one. This is good for loosening up. Variations:

(a) With a large paintbrush and one colour, make marks on paper. Change colour and repeat.

(b) Fingerpaint with opposite hand from usual one.
(c) Undertake any theme with opposite hand from usual one.

49. Left and Right Hands

Let your right hand choose a colour for itself, and the left the same. Experiment with colours, eyes closed. Open eyes and draw with both hands and both colours. Share experiences in the group.

Variation: Draw or copy a picture, first with usual hand and then with opposite one.

50. Eyes Closed

Draw or paint with your eyes closed. Good for those worried about being unable to control their drawing, or who are product oriented, as perfection is recognisably impossible. Variations:

(a) Left and Right Hands, see no. 49.
(b) Colour Exploration, see no. 37(k).

51. Straight Lines

Give participants a selection of images to choose from. Then give them a piece of A5 paper, a ruler and pencil and ask them to copy their chosen image using only the ruler and pencil, no free drawing. This can be a humorous way into discussions about control.

52. Creativity Mobilisation Technique

This is a non-verbal technique developed by Wolfgang Luthe (1976) to mobilise the brain functions to increased creativity. Detailed instructions are contained in his book *Creativity Mobilisation Technique* (see References at end of section). Here is a very brief summary:

(a) Cover 70 to 90 per cent of a double sheet of newspaper in two minutes so that it makes the biggest possible mess.
(b) Make a series of 15 such 'no thought' mess paintings.
(c) Engage in at least one painting session on four different days a week.
(d) Continue regular painting sessions for at least four to six weeks.
(e) Keep a diary of each session.

53. Wet Paper Techniques

Wet the paper and use wet paint, brushed, splattered or poured on. Watch the colours merge, and notice feelings involved. Variations:

(a) Crumple the paper as well as wetting it.
(b) Develop resulting shapes into an image.
(c) Use felt pens to draw around and between the blotches.
(d) Give titles to several quickly done blotches.

54. Ink Blots and Butterflies

Drop ink or thick blobs of paint on paper, fold in half, then unfold. Develop any image that is suggested. Variations:

(a) Give similar ink blots to different members of the group to develop and compare results.
(b) Cut out and mount a part of the blob that is particularly liked (this can help to regain a feeling of control over the process).
(c) See also nos. 32 and 33.

55. Prints and Rubbings

Use junk materials and textured objects to dip in paint and make prints, or place underneath paper and make rubbings. Variations:

(a) Use outside objects in fine weather.
(b) Group pictures of different rubbings and textures.
(c) Use prints to make a pattern.

56. Monoprints

Spread paint of a creamy consistency (e.g. Redimix paint) on a smooth surface such as stone, glass or melamine. Make a pattern or picture in the paint, with fingers, back of a paintbrush or other instrument. Press paper on top to make a print and then remove. Add more paint if necessary and repeat the process. This is useful for children (or adults) whose attempts to express ideas are frustrated by their lack of drawing ability. Variation: Use printing ink and a roller to roll it on to glass.

57. Working from Observation

Bring in things to draw from observation, then make a group picture from them, e.g. leaves, fruit, hands, tools, faces, etc. Variations:

(a) From observation, move on to questions about feelings concerned with objects.
(b) Study a flower intensely and then paint it.

58. Five Senses

Think about what colour you would associate with the present month. Then see what each of the five senses would suggest for that month. Try to relate all these aspects to yourself in a picture or poem. Particularly good for winter months when things are apparently lifeless.

59. Clothes Line

Paint on sheets of paper pegged to a clothes line. Compare this with painting on a sheet of paper on a table.

60. Just Paper

Each person in the group has one sheet of paper to use in some way to represent personal time, for 20 minutes. The paper can be torn, sellotaped, chewed, etc., but not drawn on. The process can be reflected on: by describing it; describing the product if any; noting any personal associations. Variations:

(a) Pass a piece of paper around the group, doing anything you like to it in silence, until the paper has disintegrated.
(b) Each person makes something quickly from one sheet of paper, glue and scissors.
(c) Group makes construction from rolls of newspaper, e.g. jungle and occupants.
(d) Use three pieces of paper (and glue) to:
   - get a message from the desert to someone that you're okay
   - make a present for the group;
   - make a representation of the institution.
(e) Fold and cut paper dolls, animals and other figures, evolving stories about animal families, zoos, etc. as you proceed (good for children).
(f) Tear sheets of scrap paper into pieces, then group makes picture or sculpture out of them.
(g) Use different textures and thicknesses of torn white paper to make a collage.

61. Tissue Paper

Tear up different colours of tissue paper and paste on a sheet of white paper to make abstract design. Good for people who feel they cannot draw or paint. Variations:

(a) Use only one colour of tissue paper.
(b) Cut tissue paper instead of tearing.
(c) Tissue paper work on windows.
(d) Build up tissue paper faces on paper plates.
(e) Tissue paper and wire sculptures.

62. Collage

There are many ways of experimenting with collage materials and magazine pictures, for example:

(a) Patchwork pattern quilt, see no. 102.
(b) Cut out and stick pictures of people and write down what they might be thinking or saying.
(c) Stick pieces of different fabrics on paper, then colour in between to create abstract design.
(d) Cut out pictures of landscapes and write down any associations.
(e) Use torn paper of different colours (or just plain white, see no. 60).
(f) Use natural materials.
(g) Use double-sided sellotape to make small collages on pieces of card.

63. Scratch the Surface

Cover a whole paper with colours using felt-tips or pencils. Then cover this with a layer of dark wax crayon or oil pastel. Scratch a design in the surface so that underlying colours show through.

64. Wax-resist Pictures

Draw patterns or pictures with the end of a candle (or a wax crayon) on fairly absorbent paper, then cover the paper with watery paint to make the picture appear.

65. Textures

Collect a variety of objects with different textures. After feeling them (preferably with eyes closed, maybe with the objects in a bag or box with an opening), paint a response to them or try to represent the texture in paint. This can be done in pairs or in a group.

Variation: create a mini-environment from textured materials that describe your personality, forming a 'touch box'.

66. Using Found Objects

Collect natural and artificial objects, preferably from your own environment, e.g. shells, flowers, ornaments, leaves, plants, rocks, stones, sand, water, sawdust, etc. Create a picture, collage, structure, etc. This can be on a specified theme, or left open. Variations:

(a) Outline bodies on huge piece of paper and fill in with collage of variously textured materials (see no. 129(c)).
(b) Collage from different kinds of crackers or pasta.

67. Junk Sculptures

Similar to no. 66, but using piles of assorted rubbish. There are many different ways of using rubbish:

(a) Make puppets (this can be extended to plays, puppet shows and acting).
(b) Group sculpture from scrap wood, newspaper rolls or other materials.
(c) Use cardboard boxes piled up to make totem poles and paint them.
(c) Landscape on large board.
(d) Mobiles.
(e) Work with semi-precious junk, e.g. pearls, glitter, etc.
(f) Make a particular object.

68. Nature and Beach Sculptures

Work outside gathering natural objects – twigs, stones, feathers, berries, etc. – to make individual or group sculptures. A beach is a specially good place for doing this, with sand, shells, stones of different colours, seaweed, driftwood and 'found objects' available. Many of the themes in the rest of this book can be used. Make sure that you respect protected habitats and do not pull up plants or break off living tree branches. It can be useful to take photos as the artworks are usually very impermanent.

69. Mixed Materials

Divide into small groups. Each small group is given an envelope of mixed materials (e.g. large paper, tissue paper, coloured sticky squares, drinking straws, paper strengtheners, coloured sellotape, etc.) to make a picture or object connected with a particular theme, for example, transport. Good for mixed groups of adults and children.

70. Work with Clay

There are very many ways of working with clay, for example:

(a) Getting to know it as a material – feeling, pressing, squeezing, shaping, etc; using all the senses to experience it.
(b) Make ball of clay into something with eyes closed.
(c) Hold the clay for five minutes and notice thoughts and feelings.
(d) Describe clay creation in first person.
(e) Making impressions on clay with other implements.
(f) Specified theme, e.g. individual houses for group street scene.
(g) Making simple slab pots and thumb pots.
(h) Using glazes.

71. Sand Play

Use sandbox and miniature figures of animals and people to portray situations and tell stories. Useful for children and others with communication difficulties; can be used to relive life conflicts in imaginative play.

72. Letting Off Steam

This can be encouraged with certain materials, if freely available, for example:

(a) Smashing up wood offcuts, banging nails.
(b) Large-scale Work, see no. 46.
(c) Junk Sculptures, see no. 67.
(d) Clay work, thumping and wedging it.
(e) Creativity Mobilisation Technique, see no. 52.
(f) Newspaper sculpture involving tearing and sticking, see no. 60(c) and (f).
(g) Paper techniques, see no. 60(a) and (g).
(h) Sand Play, see no. 71.

73. Working with Tactile Materials

Provide a variety of tactile materials, e.g. shaving cream, soap bubbles, sand, rice, beans, cereal, water, etc. Experiment with materials and notice the different qualities. Good for people with autistic spectrum disorders, attention difficulties and learning disabilities.

74. Papier-mâché

Make up about half a packet of good quality wallpaper paste in a bucket, and fill with strips of torn (not cut) newspaper to soak. Use the strips in moulds to make models (first grease with Vaseline). Allow a few days for papier-mâché to dry, then paint. Particularly useful for:

(a) Masks, modelled over plasticine or clay, or over a balloon (which is then 'popped').
(b) Puppets.
(c) Models of all kinds.

75. Playdough

Useful cheap modelling material, especially for young children, as it is edible (though very salty) and can be made into play food. After making it, keep in plastic bag or box in refrigerator. There are several recipes. Here are two slightly different ones:

(a) Mix 2 cups plain flour, ¾ cup salt, 1 tbsp oil, ½ cup water to consistency of pastry. The amount of water may need to be varied according to flour. Food colouring or powder paint can be added.
(b) Boil 1 tbsp oil and 4 (or more) tbsp water. Add this to 1 cup plain flour, 2 tbsp salt, 2 tsp cream of tartar and food colouring or powder paint. (The heat helps to bind the dough and the cream of tartar helps the playdough to keep longer and gives it a smoother feel.)

There are further recipes for different kinds of playdough on an information sheet from Re-Create (Cardiff Play Resource Centre), Ely Bridge Industrial Estate, Wroughton Place, Cardiff, South Wales CF5 4AB. Tel: 02920 578100. Fax: 02920 578110. E-mail: danny@re-create.co.uk. Website: www.re-create.co.uk.

76. Slime

Very popular with children. In separate containers, mix (1) in large container: 5 tbsp PVA glue and 1 tbsp glycerine (mix very thoroughly) (2) 150 ml (7 tbsp) very hot water and food colouring (3) 150 ml (7 tbsp) very hot water and 2 tsp borax. Add (2) to (1), mix thoroughly, then add (3), stirring while adding – this causes gelling. Mix until all fluid is absorbed and gelling is complete – slime will come away from sides of container. Ready when cool. If it becomes sticky after use, return to fridge to cool.

77. Creative Play with Food

Make or decorate biscuits with faces and work out dialogues before eating them up. Variations:

(a) Use other kinds of food connected together with toothpicks or cocktail sticks.
(b) Use dried pasta, lentils and beans of different kinds to create a collage.

78. Other Techniques

There is a great variety of materials and techniques that can be used in a creative way to stimulate the imagination. Here are some:

(a) Plaster of Paris, e.g. landscape, sand castings, sculptures, carvings. The plaster can be poured into an old carton to set, and the box then removed, to give a lump for carving; or it can be spread on chicken wire to make larger structures. Plaster sets very quickly and Polyfilla can sometimes be used if slower setting is desired. Plaster-impregnated bandages are quick and easy to use.
(b) Silkscreen printing, e.g. designs made from newspapers.
(c) Butterfly paintings and potato printing – see also nos. 54 and 55.
(d) Scratchboard pictures.
(e) Marbling.
(f) Abstract sculpture from wood offcuts and other materials.
(g) Batik and fabric printing.
(h) Tie-and-dye T-shirts and materials.
(i) Using fabric paints on T-shirts, baseball caps, etc.
(j) Candle making.
(k) Lanterns.
(l) Lino cuts.
(m) Pin-and-thread pictures.
(n) Kite making.
(o) Balloon masks from papier-mâché over balloons, see no. 74.
(p) Blowing paint through straws.
(q) Mosaics.
(r) Making stencils.
(s) String prints: dip string in paint, place on paper, fold paper and withdraw string while pressing down paper.
(t) Medicine wheels in the Native American/First Nations traditions (for details see Barber 2002).

References

Barber, V. (2002) *Explore Yourself Through Art: Creative Projects to Promote Personal Insight, Growth and Problem-solving*, London: Carroll & Brown.

Luthe, W. (1976) *Creativity Mobilisation Technique*, New York: Grune and Stratton.

C Concentration, dexterity and memory

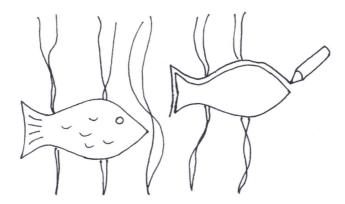

Many of these activities try to increase or maintain skills of concentration, dexterity and memory. They can be useful learning activities for children and people with learning disabilities, and for long-term patients/clients being rehabilitated to leave an institution after many years. Some of them are also useful for elderly people with dementia problems, in helping them to retain their hold on 'reality' (especially if they have to live in an institution). Even more important, they can use experiences people may have had during their lives and reaffirm their personal value in remembering what they have done.

79. Planning a Garden

Useful for those who have done a lot of gardening. Plan a garden, using drawing, painting and collage, etc.

80. Domestic Animals Mural

Using prepared templates, everyone draws his or her own version, paints and cuts out. These can then be fitted into prepared spaces on a mural and the background painted in.

81. Shelves

Using prepared paper with shelves drawn on it, imagine it as a larder and decide what to stock it with. Variations:

(a) Garden shed.
(b) Tool cupboard.
(c) Table top – what sort of meal?
(d) Washing line – what is hanging out?
(e) Shop window – what is in it?

82. Shops and Categories

Provide each member of the group with a sheet of blank paper with a different shop heading, e.g. shoe shop, grocer, garage, baker, etc. Then 'stock' the shops with appropriate articles, either drawn or cut from magazines. Variations:

(a) Head each sheet with a different colour and stick on articles of the correct colour.
(b) Each sheet headed sport, cookery and other activities.
(c) Other categories, e.g. furniture, clothes, etc.

83. Breakfast Table

Table is covered with a sheet of paper and real things – such as a teapot, toast, etc. Imagine a fantasy meal. Draw what you would like to have for breakfast on paper, using the real objects to draw around or copy if needed. Group works all around the table.
    Variation: Use cardboard cut-outs if real things not available.

84. Daily Details

Draw or cut out pictures of daily life, e.g. recent meals, events, people, clothes, etc., remembering and talking about details in the process.

85. Clothes

Photocopy a magazine portrait high up on a piece of paper. Draw rest of person in any clothes you wish. Variation: Draw own clothing from memory.

86. Houses

Supply outlines of a house for people to fill in with whatever details they want, and add further items and figures if desired. (This may lead to discussion of families and people at home.)

87. National Flags

Have available copies of various national flags to colour in. Members of the group choose the ones they want and may make associations with them. (Good for groups of elderly people who may have visited other countries, e.g. in wartime. Also for groups with a mixture of cultural backgrounds.)

88. Map-making

Draw bus, ambulance, walking or cycling routes to school, club, hospital, day centre, etc., or to any other place of interest.

89. Imaginary Traffic System

Using a collection of miniature cars, draw a large road system of a town, putting in other buildings, etc.

90. Objects

Divide a sheet of paper into, say, eight boxes, each with a different heading, e.g. a bird, a chair, a car, an animal. Group members then draw or stick an appropriate picture in each box.

91. Fruit, Flowers and Leaves

Draw or trace around leaves, flowers, fruit, found objects, etc. Paint and cut out. Make into collage as a group. Variation: Combined murals of butterflies, fish, sunflowers, etc.

92. Environments

Cut out a magazine figure and then fill in the environment around it.

93. Flower Collages

Make individual flower collages in polystyrene dishes. Display collages as a group. Variation: Use other themes for individual panels, see no. 264(a).

94. Experiences

Discuss experiences of, for example, seeing a rainbow. Then try to capture memory of this by painting rainbow, trees, hills, clouds, rain, etc. Can be applied to any experience likely to be common to the group, e.g. a recent outing.

95. Four Seasons

Take four differently coloured large sheets of paper and ask the group to choose which colour will be for each of the four seasons. Then cut out magazine pictures and stick on appropriate sheet of paper.

96. Natural Objects

Use natural objects as stimulation for discussion, painting murals.

97. Windows

Adaptation of no. 179(a). Have a variety of 'windows'. Draw view through window and what is in room (looking in or out).

98. Templates

Provide templates. Then the group uses them to draw around on card, cut out and stick on murals, e.g. Festival Themes, see no. 113.

99. Stencils

Similar to templates, but people draw inside the shape. Can also be used to apply paint to murals and for making repeating patterns.

100. Initials Design

Write your initials and make a design out of it. Variations:

(a) Use your name or nickname.
(b) Repeat each letter upside down and look at patterns and spaces made by shapes. Develop into a design.

101. Circle Patterns

Have prepared a large circle divided into segments like an orange. Group starts at the middle and works outwards, producing patterns of colour, shape, line, etc. (can also stick things on). Variation: use any other shape broken down into smaller shapes, see no. 264(b), (c), (d).

102. Patchwork Pattern Quilt

Cut out lots of 'patchwork' shapes from coloured paper and magazines. Then group members create their own pattern of 'quilt' from the pieces.
    Variation: create a large 'quilt' by everyone working on the same pattern.

103. Weaving Patterns

Weave a pattern with coloured strips of paper, working out own pattern.

104. Faces

Using prepared circles, draw faces on circles. Variations:

(a) If this is too difficult, make a stencil.
(b) Different kinds of faces: a funny face, a sad face, a silly face, etc.

105. Cut-out Shapes

Cut out shapes of people, men and women (or have them prepared) and fill them in using any desired medium. Variations:

(a) Butterfly shapes.
(b) Animal shapes.

106. Gifts

Make or draw something you would like to give to someone.

D   General themes

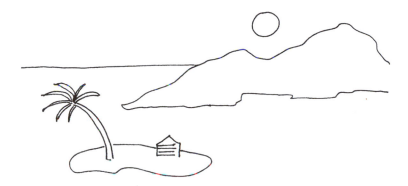

There are many themes which, although general rather than personal, can enable people to bring out important feelings in the process of painting and subsequent discussion.

107. Making and Decorating Folders

This is a good activity for a first session, when participants may be feeling nervous and apprehensive about a group. Making and decorating a folder can be a low-key way to start interacting with other group members. It also provides a safe place for future pictures to be stored.

108. Four Elements Picture Series

This series based on the four ancient elements of air, earth, fire and water. Paint 24 pictures on the themes below, each on a separate sheet:

(a) *Earth series*: cave – hut – house – courtyard – field – earth.
(b) *Water series*: spring – brook – river – lake – sea – water.
(c) *Air series*: breath – wind – storm – cloud – sky/heaven – air.
(d) *Fire series*: torch – fireplace – lamp – hearth/fire – light – fire.

These can be used as discussion points, comparing pictures of same series and comparing how different people have interpreted the theme. Some people will find that they have more affinity to one series than others and this can be a basis for discussion.

Variation: Choose only one theme (earth, water, air, fire) and do a painting on any aspect of this theme.

109. Appreciating the Elements

Think in turn about each of the elements – earth, air, fire, water. Pick one to focus on and try to experience it in a safe way. Then try to represent your feelings about this element in colours, shapes and textures, or use collage. Variations:

(a) Pick the element closest to your temperament and an opposite one. Make a picture containing both of them – use art materials and/or collage and objects.
(b) Combine the elements into separate pictures of the four seasons, or do one picture containing all four seasons.

110. House – Tree – Person

Draw a house, a tree and a person (or face). Or select one of these and set it for a group. Variations:

(a) Add landscape.
(b) Describe each one in the first person.
(c) Paint your home, or an ideal house, or an ideal island.

111. Free Painting

Paint a picture in 15 to 20 minutes. Show it to the group and say as much as you want to say. No analysis. This gives people who are prepared to share their personal feelings the space and 'permission' to do so.

112. Discussion Topic

Use a theme that has arisen from group discussion as the theme of artwork, either individual or group.

113. Festival Themes

There are many possibilities for personal work or for groupwork that can use particular festivals as starting points, for example:

(a) Celebration of festivals, e.g. Chanucah, Chinese New Year, Christmas, Diwali, Id and others. This can be done in individual or group pictures.
(b) Exploring the symbols involved in festivals.
(c) Exploring food and its place in different cultures, especially at festivals.
(d) Practical projects such as decorations for festivals.
(e) Celebration of different seasons, e.g. spring, in group pictures.
(f) New Year resolutions.
(g) Mammoth birthday card for a member of the group.
(h) Posters for events or to get over ideas.
(i) Jumble sale – drawings of rubbish.

Even though most of these themes celebrate joyful events, they may also bring back memories of happier times. Thus they may reinforce present feelings of isolation and depression, especially if people are in institutions. It is important to be aware of this.

114. Eggs and Wishes

Large plastic or cardboard egg shapes that can be opened into two halves are needed for this. Members of the group write private wishes on small pieces of paper, which are then placed in the eggs. The eggs are closed and covered with torn and glued pieces of tissue paper. They can remain covered or be opened at a later date.

115. Design Your Ideal Place

Design your ideal coffee shop, pub, café, restaurant or other similar place.

116. Seasons

Think about the four seasons and what they mean to you. Then try to express this through paint, clay or collage. Some possibilities are:

(a) Individual pictures for all the four seasons.
(b) A group picture showing all four seasons.
(c) Pick the season you like best/least to explore.
(d) Associate colours with each season.
(e) Find suitable collage materials and natural objects to include for each season.

117. Themes of Life

Choose a particular life theme and make a picture connected with it: for example, sex, gender, marriage, family; authority, freedom, growth, life and death; leaving, goodbye; the group, communication, problems; life, light, love; a force that affects your life strongly, etc. Topics may need some introduction to get started.

118. Choosing Pictures

Make up a collection of pictures cut out of magazines on a variety of themes – landscapes, people, situations, abstract patterns, artworks, etc. Paste them on card or put them in plastic sleeves. Ask members of the group to quietly choose one or two pictures that speak to them. Then people share their reasons for their choices. Variations:

(a) Collect postcards in the same way.
(b) Make up subsets on different themes, e.g. relationships.
(c) Ask people to choose according to a theme, e.g. one that reminds you of your childhood.

119. Memories

Focus on memories of particular events, as appropriate for the group, for example:

(a) An important journey.
(b) An important event, perhaps starting with a photo as the basis of a picture.
(c) An achievement you are proud of.
(d) A significant object in your life (ask group members to bring objects to the group).
(e) A significant object that has been in your family for generations.
(f) Important food associated with your country of origin (this can be particular fruits, vegetables or spices, or dishes made up of several ingredients).
(g) Paper plates and coloured plasticine can be used for (f).

120. Colour Associations

Associate colours with abstract states, for example:

(a) Emotions – sadness, fear, love, joy, calm, etc.
(b) Periods of your life – babyhood, childhood, etc.
(c) Seasons (see no. 116).
(d) Times of day.
(e) Psychological function – thinking, feeling, intuition, sensation, etc.

(f) Types of people – extrovert, introvert, etc.
(g) Members of your family, and other influential people.

121. Subjects to Illustrate

These can relate to personal experiences or provide a more covert way of expressing oneself. Children and adolescents can often use them in this way. There is an infinite number of such themes; here are a few:

(a) Nature – desert, mountain, rock, plants, trees, animals, birds, fish, shells.
(b) Weather – storm, thunder and lightning, sun, snow, rain, cloud, wind, fire, hot day, twilight, moonlight.
(c) Hot and cold – what makes you think of these?
(d) Water – raindrops, waterfalls, whirlpools, ripples, waves, sea, river, lake, etc.
(e) Gardens – secret gardens, mazes, labyrinths.
(f) Changed perspectives – ant's, bird's, elephant's eye view.
(g) View from a window – what's inside and what's outside?
(h) People – villain, devil, ghosts, magician, angel, witch, fairies, clown.
(i) Superheroes/heroines.
(j) Religious – images of God; good and evil; heaven and hell; spiritual experience; meditation, etc.
(k) Dreams and nightmares (see also no. 342).
(l) Group situations – fight, war, circus, fair, orchestra, etc.
(m) Fantasy – other planets, outer space, exploring a cave, character from TV or story, etc.
(n) Events – the weekend, a day trip, my day, my week, journeys made, expected or desired, etc.
(o) Model clay animals and then make an environment for them all.

122. Islands

Draw an island as if approaching it from outer space. Variations:

(a) Decide what to keep and what to change.
(b) Make it into your ideal island.
(c) Use as basis for interactive work where members of the group visit each others' islands.
(d) See also no. 260.

123. Action and Conflict Themes

These can be useful for those who cannot easily articulate their conflicts, but can depict them graphically through another situation; for instance, some children and adolescents.

(a) Graffiti on large sheets of paper.

(b) Ghosts and skeletons.

(c) Fires, e.g. ship on fire.

(d) Life on another planet.

(e) In prison (from inside or outside).

(f) 'Wanted' posters.

(g) Sport – boxing, football, etc.

(h) Storms, e.g. at sea; or stormy sky with sunny part in corner.

(i) Explosions, volcanoes, etc.

(j) Battles.

(k) Underwater pictures.

(l) Prehistoric or mythical monsters; monster inside someone's head; horrible slimy creature in mud; creating and dealing with one's own monster.

(m) Murder.

(n) Moods, e.g. mood changes; sad and miserable; angry; happy thoughts; frightened; excited; peaceful; lonely; trapped; feeling ill.

(o) Draw around hands and wrists, then add watch, rings, scars, veins, tattoos, etc.

124. Personal Experiences

Artwork around events that people have experienced, e.g. a special trip, a particular ward, etc.

Variation for children: experiences with pets and animals. This can evoke strong feelings of protectiveness, responsibility, fear or violence, according to the experience. It may be easier for some children to express their feelings about animals than about people.

E Self-perceptions

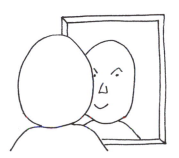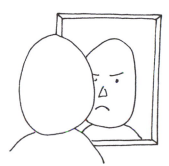

Most of this section is concerned, in a variety of ways, with how people see themselves. This can be a refreshing and reflective experience for many people, but can be too confrontational for very hurt or damaged people, who may find the less direct themes in Section D more suitable.

125. Introductions

The idea of this is to introduce yourself to the group on paper. This can be less threatening than a verbal introduction, as everyone does it at once. It can also include a variety of styles, such as including family members, hobbies, likes and dislikes, self-portraits – or be done in an abstract way using lines and colours. Additional instructions can include drawing whatever might describe yourself, including your name, etc. Variations:

(a) Make and decorate folders (see no. 107).
(b) Produce a poster for display for duration of group/conference, etc.
(c) Poster to illustrate your lifestyle for another person.
(d) Include specific attitudes, interests, characteristics, family, friends, etc.
(e) Include things you like or are good at.
(f) Use collage.

(g) Bring to first meeting of group.
(h) Personal worlds: visualise your world in colours, lines, shapes and symbols, or how you would like it to be.

126. Self-portraits: Realistic

Do a realistic portrait of yourself, in pastels, paint or clay, making sure that details, etc. are right. Variations:

(a) Self-portrait from memory – face or nude.
(b) Quick realistic portrait, in two minutes or other time limit.
(c) Clay self-portrait with eyes closed; touch face with one hand, modelling with the other.
(d) Touch face, then draw it.
(e) Draw nude figure of yourself. Then, at home, compare your drawing with what you see in mirror. (This exercise may be best done individually and then shared in the group.)
(f) Make movable clay and wire marionette to resemble self, with environment to scale. This helps to accept physical reality through transitional object.
(g) Select photograph most like oneself. Can be good for helping discussion of disabilities or disfigurements, e.g. mothers of children with disabilities.
(h) Skin colour: look at self in mirror and then match the skin colour. Good for groups of children to start discussion of race and colour issues.

127. Self-portraits: Images

Do self-portrait:

(a) How you see yourself or feel inside yourself.
(b) How others (e.g. someone close, such as family members) see you (or how you present yourself). They can be realistic or abstract.

Variations:

(a) Add a third contrast: how you would like to be seen.
(b) Use clay or collage; or mixed media.
(c) How you see yourself today/right now.
(d) Yourself as seen by sympathetic friend and by someone you dislike.
(e) As for (d), but write about yourself from these two points of view.
(f) Only do 'How I perceive myself'.

(g) Imagine piece of paper is mirror on door. What do you see (realistic, metaphorical or abstract)?
(h) Four selves – actual, perceived, ideal, future.
(i) Self box – see no. 128.
(j) Self-portrait, exaggerating how you think you look.
(k) Apply to particular roles, e.g. professional self.
(l) Make several masks to show different aspects of yourself that you show in different circumstances, and also a mask to show how you really feel.
(m) As for (l), but show all the aspects on one mask.
(n) As for (l) or (m) but use collage materials or 'media images' cut from magazine.
(o) Do this exercise in relation to race, colour, culture or gender issues. This can be used to reflect on societal stereotypes and personal reactions to them.

128. Self-portraits: Using Bags and Boxes

Use collage images to represent how you feel inside and outside yourself by using inside and outside of box, bag or other container. Variations:

(a) Symbol of important goal on top of upturned box and symbols of what you want to change on the sides of the box. (Acrylic paints, which dry very quickly, can be used to make further changes.)
(b) Outside of box showing your roles; inside of box filled with objects or pictures relating to your values, friends, family, hobbies, things important to you.
(c) Use junk materials.
(d) Use paper bags to paste pictures on outside of what you show to the world, and put inside what you keep inside.
(e) Repeat (d) above for others close to you, e.g. mother, father, spouse, children, etc. Are there similarities?
(f) Draw or paint abstract symbols on separate pieces of paper to represent your values. Put inside the bag those you always have, and outside those which apply only to your present situation.
(g) Paste outside the best things that can happen to you. Inside put a collection of your fears.
(h) Use the box to make a hidden door or gateway and build the world behind it.
(i) Use the inside of the box or bag for secrets. It is important not to put pressure on group members to disclose these, while providing an opportunity for people to do so if they want to.
(j) Start with a plan of a box to be made up, and stick personal qualities and other things on it. Then stick the box together and reflect on the relationship of the items stuck on.

(k) Use old hats (or make some from card) in the same way as boxes. Then people can wear them and see how this feels.

Figure E.1 shows a group at an alcohol unit sharing ideas on using junk materials to make self-portraits in tins and boxes.

129. Life-size Self-portraits

Pin a large roll of paper to the wall. Draw round yourself, then work on the life-size body image in any way you like. Be careful about using this exercise with groups who find touch difficult or have problems with body image. Variations:

(a) Person lies on floor and someone else traces round on paper.
(b) Life-size body image of how you use the different parts of your body to communicate how you feel.
(c) Trace body outline, name parts and fill in with colours or collage materials, or with what is going on inside you, physically and mentally, or with lines of energy.
(d) Draw silhouettes of body parts, cut out and arrange on a mural.
(e) Life-size portrait of what it is like to be yourself right now.
(f) Talk to your outline; imagine yourself in front of you.
(g) Choose a section of body image to explore in another painting.
(h) See if a parent is associated with any particular part of the body.
(i) Fill in with own likeness, e.g. hair and clothes worn (good for children).
(j) Make life-size model to act as 'other self'.
(k) Use full-length mirror (good for children).
(l) Locate places of stress inside body and add external stress factors.
(m) Mark emotional injuries at different ages on relevant parts of body.
(n) Use exercise as basis for expressing feelings about sexuality (only do this with an established group).

130. Hands and Feet

Draw round hands and feet and make them into a picture. Reflect on what they do for you. Variation: use hand and foot prints in paint.

131. 3-D Self-portraits

Build a representation of yourself in 3-D, using junk materials. Variations:

(a) Self box (see no. 128). Or use junk materials inside and outside box.
(b) Work with large lump of clay in any way, without trying to make a model. When finished, place on table to reflect where you would feel comfortable if the clay were you.

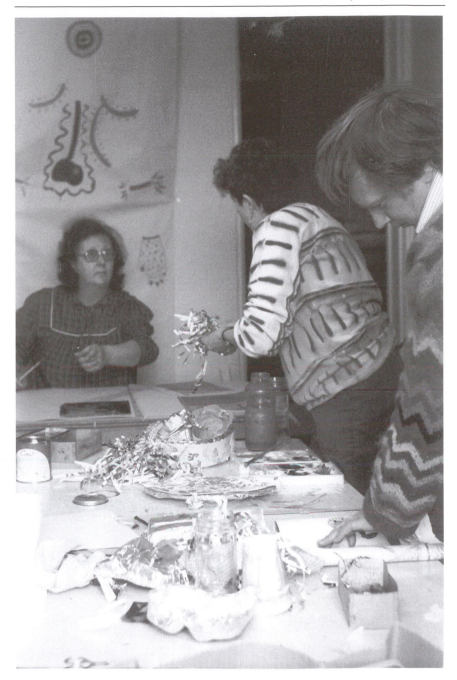

Figure E.1 Self-portraits in boxes, using junk materials – alcohol unit
Source: Photograph by Paul Curtis

(c) Make a movable clay marionette to resemble yourself.

(d) Make a relief clay portrait inside a shoe box; let it dry and paint it.

(e) Eyes closed, visualise a round ball changing into a realistic or abstract image of yourself. Then create image with hands. Open eyes to finish off.

(f) Clay hands: roll some clay into a ball and press down with one hand to make a handprint. Scratch a symbol which represents something friendly about you. Repeat for a hand of a person you like and arrange two hands in suitable positions.

(g) See also nos. 126(c) and 127(b).

132. Sexuality and Gender

Use paint, crayons, clay or collage to express thoughts and feelings about your sexuality and/or gender. Variations:

(a) Chart your awareness of the development of your sexuality.

(b) Chart the development of your awareness of gender differences.

(c) Concentrate on celebrating positive aspects.

(d) Attributes of your ideal woman/man.

(e) Choose a character from life or fiction to use with (c).

(f) Group pictures on essence of manhood and womanhood. It can be interesting to have two smaller groups, one working on each of these.

This can bring up difficult feelings, so be aware of your group before exploring this topic.

133. Celebrating Diversity

Make an individual picture celebrating any aspect of yourself, such as race, colour, culture, heritage. Use any art materials or a collage of positive images. Variations:

(a) Positive qualities from family and ancestors, things you are proud of about your heritage.

(b) Group members talk about where they have come from and then do some artwork on any aspect of this.

(c) Do a group picture, either from the start or putting together individual contributions.

(d) Work with black and white paint and reflect on the associations, thoughts and feelings that come up.

(e) Make a paper 'patchwork quilt' of all the elements in your cultural heritage. Many people feel themselves to be members of more than one culture and this is a way of expressing these identities.

(f) Create a racial/cultural map of all the events and people making up your current identity.

(g) Using (f) as a basis, imagine finding yourself in a foreign land with unfamiliar language, environment, customs, etc. Explore your feelings and create an image. What aspects of your original cultural map would help you cope with your new situation?

(h) Make two pictures about your national/cultural identity, one which might seem threatening to another group, one which is non-threatening. Discuss with others.

(i) Explore flags, emblems and symbols denoting cultural heritage.

Extend these exercises to other groups, e.g. gay and lesbian identities, class, gender, etc.

134. Masks

Make a mask of yourself using thin card or a paper plate. Put it on and act the role your mask suggests. Variations:

(a) Make a mask to express a particular emotion – see also no. 162.

(b) Make up/use stories which involve masks.

(c) Link up with no. 127, masks of how you see yourself and how others see you.

(d) See also no. 153 Public and Private Masks; no. 154 Good and Bad, masks that represent ideal and unacceptable sides of yourself.

(e) Mask of a side of yourself that people do not usually see that you would like to wear.

(f) Make half-face masks (top and/or bottom) and see how they feel.

(g) Use plaster of Paris bandages to make face masks, allowing space for eyes, nose and mouth. (Put vaseline on face before doing this.) Be careful with people who do not like being touched, but sometimes they are happy to join in the mask making.

(h) See also nos. 184 and 185 for other uses of masks.

135. Body Armour

Create armour for different aspect of your personality, positive and negative; e.g. shield for strength, spear for anger. Wear the pieces and talk about them to others.

Variation: If you are facing a challenge in your life, make the armour you need to help you through this.

136. Names

Draw images of:

(a) your nickname when a child;
(b) your proper name;
(c) a fantasy name.

Variations:

(a) Pick a name for yourself according to your feelings and embellish it in some way.
(b) Using opposite hand from usual, write your name:

   • backwards
   • forwards to fill the whole space
   • very slowly.

(c) Combine with other exercises about yourself.
(d) Use your initials to make a pattern.
(e) Add to your name any cultural associations and meanings from your background.

Names and initials can bring up strong feelings, especially if they remind people of others in their lives and circumstances of pain or distress.

137. Badges and Symbols

Find and draw your own symbol. If this is difficult, think of other everyday visual symbols first. Variations:

(a) Develop your own symbol for use on a personal shield.
(b) Make up a strip cartoon using your own symbol.
(c) Make a badge for yourself to represent a quality of yours that you are proud of.
(d) Make up a symbol for a personal T-shirt.
(e) Make up a slogan to go with your symbol.
(f) Make own coat of arms with motto, symbol, epitaph, etc.
(g) Model your own personal plaque using clay or other modelling material.

138. Metaphorical Portraits

Draw yourself as some kind of object. The choice of object can be left open to see what is produced, or it can be specified: e.g. draw yourself as a house, tree, animal, food, island, colours and shapes, building, flower, plant, meal, water, tree or landscape. If appropriate, include a setting (garden, fruit bowl, landscape, etc.). Variations:

(a) After drawing the object, talk about it in the first person, act as if you were that object.
(b) What object (animal, building, etc.) would you like to be?
(c) What object (animal, building, etc.) would you be if reincarnated?
(d) Draw yourself as an object that represents how you are feeling today.
(e) Draw yourself as the animal (etc.) you would:

- most like to be
- least like to be.

(f) Draw yourself as an object and as an animal, on opposite sides of the paper. (Do these relate to how you are treated by others, or how you relate to others?)
(g) Dynamic metaphors. For example, using an image of a developing seed, illustrate a point of growth which relates to you, noting reactions to process of growth.
(h) Choose several colours and make a drawing that represents yourself.
(i) For people who tend to isolate themselves, ask for a setting to be included.

139. Advertisements

Draw/paint an advertisement for yourself. This can involve 'selling oneself' and bring up negative feelings from lack of self-esteem, and can also involve thinking about the sort of people to be attracted by the advertisement. Variations:

(a) After each person has finished, others in the group add to each advertisement aspects missed out.
(b) Advertisement to sell you as a friend, worker, parent, etc.
(c) Write or draw advertisements for others.
(d) Depict a department store displaying your personal qualities. After this, a 'shopping trip' to select wares from others' stores to make another picture.
(e) Focus on achievements.

140. Lifeline

Draw your life as a line, journey, roadmap or river. Put in images and events along the way, drawn and/or written. Variations:

(a) Select one section of your line and draw an image.
(b) Choose one part only to depict as a line, or a particular aspect, e.g. friends, work life, sexual life, cultural awareness, etc.
(c) Use sections labelled 'past', 'present' and 'future'.
(d) Draw your life as a maze, if appropriate.
(e) Use the whole piece of paper to depict your lifetime, or use a roll of paper.
(f) Use different sorts of lines/colours for different experiences.
(g) Lifeline as a spiral, starting from birth.
(h) Continue lifeline into future.
(i) Illustrate your life story with images from magazines.
(j) Draw map of important things, places and people in your life.
(k) Cartoon strip of your life.
(l) Place special emphasis on where you are going.
(m) Survey past artwork from specific period.
(n) Include barriers and detours and role play overcoming these.
(o) Story of how you came to particular situation, e.g. prison, hospital, in trouble, etc.
(p) Draw your life as some kind of transport, e.g. bike, car, bus, train or boat, etc. Include yourself and other important people.

141. Snakes and Ladders

Devise your own game of snakes and ladders, using events and images from your life as snakes and ladders. Play your game with another person.

142. Past, Present and Future

This is another view of the same theme as no. 140, but in more distinct blocks. Draw images of your past, present and hoped for future. Variations:

(a) Concentrate on future only. Visualise the future in images – immediate future, five years, ten years ahead.
(b) Concentrate on the present, here-and-now experiences.
(c) Use images from magazines.
(d) Your life at particular moments, e.g. ten years ago, one year from now, etc., or at particular ages.
(e) Past, present and future self-images. Explore any conflicts of content.
(f) Concentrate on particular aspects of future, e.g. what job you would like, what sort of house, etc.
(g) Imagine yourself at a crossroads. What are your alternative directions?
(h) Decisions made/to be made.
(i) Changes and hopes for the New Year (etc.).

(j) Things that may be difficult in the near future.

(k) Scale of states from 'ideal' to 'rock bottom'. Mark where you are now and the steps needed to move upwards. Perhaps link with no. 140 (Lifeline) to see what patterns have influenced you.

(l) Yourself at this moment in the context of past and future life.

(m) Personal coat of arms with spaces for specific information, e.g. hope for next year.

(n) Feelings of leaving one experience and going to another.

(o) Ideal world.

(p) Where I came from, where I am now and where I am going.

(q) Unfinished business.

(r) Regrets and how you would have liked things to be.

(s) Losses you have suffered in your life and what you would like to find in the future. See also no. 150.

(t) People important to you, or important in the past.

(u) Before and after: draw yourself or your life and how you felt before and after a particular event, e.g. accident, becoming ill, getting married, moving house, etc.

(v) Do separate pictures for past, present and future. Then place them on the floor like stepping stones. Walk from one to the other, noticing your feelings as you do so.

(w) Bridge from past to future, with what you are leaving behind and what you are moving on to.

143. Life Collage

Pick out from magazines pictures that are relevant to your life (ten minutes), cut out words (five minutes) and put together into collage representing your life (30 minutes). Variations:

(a) Cut out a headline relevant to you and your life.

(b) Take out the contents of your pocket/handbag and arrange the objects according to the emotional distance from you and each other, to make a pattern of your life.

(c) Draw your concerns and arrange on paper to form a 'life-space' picture.

(d) Pick out three to five pictures that make a statement about you, or show things you are willing to share.

144. Life Priorities Collage

On a large piece of paper, paint three horizontal bands of colour to represent far, middle and near distances. Then cut out or draw pictures to represent different aspects of your work, family and social life (or just one of these, e.g. social life). Stick these pictures on to the appropriate band of colour with blu-tak or other removable adhesive. When you have finished, reflect on the results and move pictures around until the whole feels 'comfortable'. Useful in trying to reassess priorities.

145. Aspects of Self

Make a map with yourself in the centre and place different aspects of yourself around the centre in relationship to one another, bearing in mind distance, size, etc. Variations:

(a) Map of important things, places and people in your life, in relation to yourself.
(b) Three bands of colour for spiritual, mental and physical aspects. Discuss colour, textures, widths of bands in group, or pair up with someone with similar pattern.
(c) Mandala (centred image) of different aspects of self from centre outwards (see also no. 349).
(d) 'Community' of selves. Depict your various roles (e.g. car driver, parent, etc.) as a community on one piece of paper.

146. Recent Events

Think back over last week/night and represent something that made you happy, and then something upsetting.
    Variation: Depict events of last week in strip cartoon form.

147. Childhood Memories

Draw your first or early memory, a childhood memory, or a memory which made a deep impression. These themes often bring up hurts from childhood that people have been unaware of and can be difficult to deal with. It is important to allow enough time for discussion of these. Variations:

(a) A warm or happy childhood memory and an unhappy one.
(b) A good memory and a bad one.
(c) An embarrassing moment.
(d) An important object from your childhood, e.g. a toy, container, book, etc.
(e) Yourself as a child.
(f) Memories associated with strong feelings.
(g) Paint first memory with other hand from the usual one.
(h) Talk and paint like children of six to ten years, using fingerpainting.
(i) Write name in paint, first with right hand and then with left hand.

(j) Things you were not allowed in childhood. (Are these the things you feel most guilty about as an adult?)

(k) Draw memory as if at that age.

(l) 'Melting mirror' – a technique to reach back to childhood in imagination. As you look at yourself in a mirror, it seems to melt and the image wavers. When it settles it reveals you as a child in a room in your house (settle on any age that seems to suggest itself). Imagine the room and a conversation between you and your child self. What does the child say to you? What do you reply? Paint the situation. Then see if there are any messages in it for you now.

(m) First memory of separation and present-day hellos and goodbyes. (Are there any connections?) This can bring up strong feelings.

148. Life Review

Draw or paint significant memories from your life. This can be useful for elderly people or those at a crossroads, in reviewing their lives. Some examples:

(a) Images from childhood, adolescence and adulthood.

(b) A good memory and a bad one.

(c) An embarrassing moment.

(d) Memories associated with strong feelings.

(e) Important events, e.g. weddings, births, deaths, leaving home, migration, etc.

(f) Important groups of people, e.g. family, friends, village, workmates, religious groups, etc.

(g) City scenes and country scenes.

(h) Use old family photographs to build up picture album of life and events.

(i) Important ingredients of life, e.g. pets, houses, job, hobbies, activities specially enjoyed. Any of these can also be developed into longer projects.

(j) Daily life now and several years ago, and associated feelings.

(k) Depict family, friends, etc. with whom you have left something unsaid or unfinished. Add what you would have wished to say or do.

(l) Pass round objects from a previous era or another life, such as household items, tools, etc. These can be a stimulus for many memories. (Members of the group may be able to contribute objects for this.) If there are regrets or trauma associated with the transition (e.g. refugees), care will be needed to work with this sensitively.

(m) Life review in stages.

149. Life Stage Concerns

Use life stage concerns as themes, e.g. adolescence, middle age, etc. Ask about the concerns in a general way: for example, What are adolescents concerned about? What do girls your age find most annoying?

150. Losses

Draw a picture or abstract symbol of someone or something which has gone. Variations:

(a) Feelings surrounding this event.
(b) See also no. 197, Bereavement Issues and no. 284, Bereavement Balloons.

This theme may be very cathartic and should be used with care, especially if people have suffered recent significant losses, but it may provide a valuable starting point for sharing important feelings. It can also be useful for older adults suffering more gradual losses of physical abilities. See also comments for no. 148, Life Review.

151. Luggage Labels

Use luggage labels to write your name and destination (real, metaphorical or fantasy) on one side, and draw your personal baggage on the other side.

152. Secrets and Privacy

Depict realistically or abstractly three things:

(i)   to be shared by the group
(ii) perhaps to be shared
(iii) not to be shared.

In the discussion, people may decide after all to share (ii) and (iii), but there should be no pressure to do so. Variations:

(a) The private you and the shared you.
(b) The part you show to the world, and the part you do not show.
(c) See also no. 128, Self-portraits: Using Boxes and Bags, especially (i).
(d) Being alone; being with others.
(e) Masks, or series of masks, for any of above. No pressure to share private masks. See also no. 153.

153. Public and Private Masks

Using a prepared mask, draw the face that you 'put on' in the morning for the world to see. Then draw a more private face that not many people see. Hold up each over your face and talk about yourself with your different 'faces' on. This exercise allows people to choose their own level of privacy to expose, which should be respected. Most people find it threatening to expose themselves too deeply in a group.

154. Good and Bad

Depict your good side and bad side, things you like and dislike about yourself, or things you would like to keep or change; or strengths and weaknesses, etc. Variations:

(a) Clay shapes of aspects liked and disliked.
(b) Masks that represent ideal and unacceptable sides.
(c) Ideal self and real self.
(d) Look at negative and positive aspects in a painting and have a conversation with both parts.
(e) Changes made and to be made.
(f) Use paper bag for faces on both sides.

155. Positive Qualities

Make a set of cards with positive qualities written on them, e.g. resourceful, friendly. Ask members of the group to pick three at random (unseen) and draw pictures of a time in their lives when they showed each quality. Variations:

(a) Things I am proud of.
(b) Make a Happy Box (good for children).
(c) Draw what 'respect' means to you.

156. Ideal People

Draw, paint or sculpt your ideal therapist/teacher/parent/friend, etc. What would they say and do, how would they help you, etc? Discuss the realities and recognise the space in between.

Variation: imagine you can ask for an extra physical attribute to be superhuman. Draw what it might be (e.g. an extra pair of eyes). Discuss what this would enable you to do.

157. Conflicts

Depict any kind of conflict, external or internal. Or conflicting parts of your personality. Variations:

(a) Animated metaphor of parts of personality in a cartoon strip.
(b) Depict any present conflict and your parents sorting out their conflicts.
(c) Draw or model two opposing aspects of your personality. Give them voices and make up a dialogue (see also no. 358).
(d) Paint or draw a conflict and its ideal solution.
(e) Paint or draw a conflict with two sides. Then, looking at it pictorially, pick elements from both sides and make a new picture. See if this has any messages for dealing with the original conflict. See also no. 239, for doing this exercise with a partner.
(f) Depict split feelings and ambivalence.
(g) Use clay.

158. Anger

Draw an outline of a person and then mark on it the physical symptoms of your anger, using colours and lines that fit the symptoms. There is a series of exercises about anger in Chapter 6, Examples 7 and 14.

159. Problems

Portray any current problem, especially if it is persistent or recurrent. Then do another picture, or a collage of any benefits of having the problem. Variations:

(a) Portray the problem, then you overcoming the problem.
(b) Do a picture of the coping skills you have for the problem.
(c) Choose colours and shapes to depict stress. Then do the same for whatever feeling is the opposite.

160. Trunks and Dustbins

Use the metaphor of trunks and dustbins for people to put in unwanted things in their lives. A trunk can be used to store things, so that they can be shut away for now but accessed in the future. A dustbin can be used for things that people want to discard (either recognised as dysfunctional or as no longer necessary).

161. Empathy with Disability

Work on a picture with various restrictions, noting your feelings, practical difficulties and how you cope with them. Try any of these:

(a) Blindfolded.
(b) Restricted hearing.
(c) Use of only one hand.
(d) Use of feet.
(e) Use of mouth only.

162. Emotions

Paint different emotions and moods, using lines, shapes, textures or colours. The emotions can be chosen individually or selected by the group. Variations:

(a) Select pairs of opposites, e.g. love/hate, anger/calm, and combine into one picture.
(b) Quick abstract drawings in response to a spoken word, e.g. love, hate, anger, peace, work, family, etc.
(c) Start on even note, doodling with crayon, then express strong negative emotion (e.g. anger), then finish in opposite mood.
(d) Paint as many emotions as you can think of.
(e) Select one emotion for a theme painting, e.g. fear, anger.
(f) Make a mask to express particular emotion.
(g) Mark different emotions in circle and put colours to them. Week by week take each one and do a separate picture.
(h) Draw objects associated with pleasant or unpleasant feelings or memories.
(i) Situations involving other people in which you have felt angry, anxious and peaceful.
(j) Paint a 'crazy' picture (whatever your perception of 'crazy' is).
(k) Cut out magazine pictures for particular emotions, e.g. angry people, and imagine what they might be saying.
(i) Use clay to express strong feelings and make an 'angry object', using tools to cut, hammer, bash clay, etc.

163. Feelings and Feasibility

Draw a situation that has raised strong feelings. Draw what you feel like doing. Then, after reflection, do another drawing showing a more feasible course of action.

164. Present Mood

Paint a picture of your mood or feelings at the moment. If appropriate, depict a metaphor, e.g. 'I'm all at sea', 'Everything's blank', etc. Variations:

(a) Use marks, shapes, colours to represent physical and emotional feelings of moment.
(b) Use symbol to express current mood.
(c) Use doodles.
(d) Select one or more and paint picture of 'I am', 'I feel', 'I have', 'I do'.
(e) Paint recent or recurring problem of feeling. (See also no. 162, Emotions.)
(f) Feelings of leaving one experience and going to another.
(g) Use for physical pain, e.g. headache, backache, etc.
(h) Do drawing of how you feel now. Then exaggerate that feeling, or part of the drawing, into a series of further drawings.
(i) Draw a large arc and label it from 0 to 10. Then cut out pictures for each number. Can add a pointer and use to think about level of mood at any point.

165. Externalising Emotions into Characters

Take emotions or states, such as depression, feeling 'snappy', impulsive, etc. and develop them into monsters or helpful creatures, with personalities of their own. 'If impulse were a creature, what would it look like?' Draw the creature and develop activities and dialogue with other parts of the self.

166. Objects and Feelings

Look at an object (flower, leaf, shell, etc.) for two minutes. Then draw your feelings about it. Variations:

(a) Look for longer period.
(b) Use only colours, lines and shapes.
(c) Choose an object that means a lot to you.

167. Survival Needs

After an imaginative journey (see Section J) involving shipwreck on a desert island, paint a picture of your island, considering topography, means of survival, length of stay, etc. Variations:

(a) Place yourself on a desert island with the things most important for your survival. What would you leave behind?
(b) Draw all the things you need – and then all the things you want.

(c) Create your own island and indicate the activities and people there.
(d) Use a folder as a 'suitcase' to take a few important things if home were endangered. Put address on it. Useful especially if this resonates with people's (or their relatives') experience, e.g. refugees.

168. Wishes

Paint one wish, three or five wishes. (More wishes demands greater imagination and can stretch people beyond conventional wishes.) Variations:

(a) A journey you would like.
(b) Where I would like to be right now.
(c) Fantasy adventure in cartoon strip, including yourself.
(d) What would you do with £1 million?
(e) What would you have from a fantasy shop window?
(f) What would you like to find in a treasure chest?
(g) What would you like to find in an attic (and put in it)?
(h) Your hero/heroine.
(i) Illustrate an important hope and fear.
(j) A present you would like to receive (or give) and from (or to) whom?
(k) You are crossing a river. What is on the other side?
(l) You are a seed beginning to grow. What is the environment?
(m) Imagine a refuge which is a secure tranquil place. What is it like and who is with you? What are the stresses and strains you would like to escape from?

169. Fears

Paint worst fear or one fear, three fears or five fears (see comment under no. 168). Variations:

(a) Imagine you are hiding – where and from what?
(b) Threatening situations.
(c) You are adrift in a boat – what would you do?
(d) You are lost in a forest – what would you do?
(e) You are locked in a prison – how would you get out?
(f) Imagine a door or a gate – what lies behind it?

170. Spirituality

Draw or paint a picture to express something to do with your spirituality, or things you hold sacred.
   Variation: Whatever sustains you spiritually.

171. Pictorial Narratives

Explore a theme in narrative form, by telling a story in a number of frames, like a comic strip, with or without words. (It is a good idea to draw in the frames first or beforehand, e.g. divide the paper into nine equal rectangles or squares.) The story can occupy as many frames as seems appropriate. Some examples:

(a) Tell a story about the journey of your life/your life script.
(b) Tell a story about what makes you tense/afraid.
(c) You are lost/adrift in a boat/in prison – what happens?
(d) Tell a story about where you would wish to be in life.
(e) Tell a story about the benefits of work, other than money.
(f) Tell a story of what happens when you come to the end of a journey.
(g) You are on a trip in an isolated area when your car gets stuck. What would you do?

Many of the themes in this section can be adapted to this form, which encourages people to put themselves in the story as the central character (although not always) and 'own' their actions and feelings. It is also a manageable and culturally accepted visual form for those who find the idea of 'painting pictures' strange and difficult. It can be particularly useful in helping people to come to terms with life crises and plan viable futures. For children, it can be useful to make comic strips (or series of stick-on labels) about people or animals who undergo similar experiences or emotions to their own, for example:

(h) Make up a picture story of a little dog who got lost.

It can also be helpful for the therapist or facilitator to suggest an appropriate 'happy ending'. For further details, see Donnelly (1983).

(i) Comic strips are useful for looking at the lead-up to a criminal offence, an angry outburst or other crises. Group members can discuss them in pairs and help each other look at what people can do to prevent a recurrence (see Liebmann 1990).

172. Likes and Dislikes

Depict a person you dislike and how she/he sees you. Then do the same for a person you like. Possibly compare qualities with yourself. Variations:

(a) Draw disliked person, then do what you will to it – tear up, etc.
(b) Pick out faces you like and dislike and make a collage (see also no. 175).

(c) Make clay shapes for likes and dislikes.
(d) Describe your best friend, then see how many qualities apply to you.
(e) Divide paper into six or eight sections and depict someone you admire, hate, love, pity, would like to change places with, who is often on your mind, etc.
(f) Draw something you like about yourself or are proud of.
(g) Pick out pictures of same sex people you admire and make a collage.

173. Friendship Series

There are many possible aspects of friendship. Here are some possibilities:

(a) A friend from the past.
(b) The qualities of a friend.
(c) A future friend.
(d) Friendship with yourself.
(e) Draw yourself in situations with and without friends.

These all lead to discussion about friendship and sometimes loneliness issues.

174. Perceptions of Self and One Other

Draw an abstract image of yourself and one other important person. Variations:

(a) Select two coloured shapes to represent self and other.
(b) Restrict choice of other person to inside or outside group.
(c) Ideal partner and imaginary opponent.
(d) Paint from standpoint of particular role, e.g. child, parent, etc.

175. Shadow of Self

Arrange a group of cut-out photographs of faces disliked (or liked) with the most disliked (or liked) in the centre of the group. Can use Gestalt technique with result (see Part I, Chapter 2, pp. 47–9). Variations:

(a) Draw image/symbol of characteristics thought most opposed to one's own. Identify with and discuss reactions to doing so.
(b) Note characteristics of same sex persons who affect you negatively (e.g. parents, peers). Collect magazine pictures to represent these and paste on sheet with most negative central to the group. Live with collage for a week, then start dialogue with it.
(c) Synthesise negative characteristics in picture. Can use Gestalt technique with result.

(d) Draw someone you hate in his or her most vile manifestations. Afterwards, try to recognise that this is a self-portrait. This is a way to
discover unacceptable, disowned portions of the self which are
projected on to others.

176. Anima/Animus

Select magazine pictures related to both very positive and very negative
feelings towards the opposite sex. Variations:

(a) Draw images of your:

- animus and anima
- good and bad sides.

Compare and discuss, especially if rigid demarcations result.

(b) Draw person, then person of opposite sex.
(c) Draw how you imagine you would feel if you were the opposite sex.
(d) Male/female – what do you consider are their different roles/
characteristics?

177. Introvert/Extrovert

List or draw imagined qualities of person of opposite temperament to
yourself (i.e. introverts list imagined qualities of extrovert). Then paint as if
you had one or more of these qualities.

178. Personal Space

Select your own size of paper and draw yourself somewhere on it.
Variations:

(a) Choose colour and size of paper and write your name on it. Decorate
the rest if you wish.
(b) After choosing size, provide standard size paper and see if anyone asks
for larger or smaller size paper.
(c) Draw yourself in (outer) space.
(d) If the paper represents you, how much is filled by a current concern?

179. Personal Landscape

Draw a landscape (town, sea or countryside) and relate it to you personally.
Variations:

(a) Draw window of any size. Show view through window and what is in room. Realistic or abstract. (Results are sometimes looking out, sometimes looking in.)
(b) Take imaginary pictures with shoebox camera, focusing on what is significant in room.
(c) Paint yourself in a landscape.
(d) Paint an ideal or favourite place (or one disliked).

180. Safe Place

Draw, paint or model a safe place to be or hide. This can be a safe place remembered from childhood or in the current situation. This theme can be useful when there are issues about confidentiality or trust. Variations:

(a) Suggest that group members take one thing into their safe space that gives them some comfort.
(b) A safe place for a chosen animal/puppet (useful for children).

181. Personal Progression

Draw a picture that answers the question 'Who are you?' Try to make progressively more meaningful pictures each time in answer to the question. Write a description of each picture.

182. Time Progression

Portray the people in your life who influence you, during the first week of therapy, a course, etc. Repeat three or four months later.

183. Personal Time

Do a picture showing what you usually do in a typical day/24 hours/week.

184. Before and After Masks

Members of the group draw or paint a mask as they arrive at the group, then put it on one side, face down. At the end of the session, they draw another mask, then compare the two and discuss any changes in feelings and perceptions.

185. Mask Diary

Similar to no. 184, but 'before' and 'after' masks are drawn throughout the life of the group and put away in a folder. Towards the end of the sessions, they are spread out and each person shares their journey through their masks. In an ongoing group, a good time to share the masks would be after five to eight weeks.

186. Reviewing Artwork

Look back at paintings and other artwork done over a period of time and notice any patterns or recurring themes. Also make any new connections that seem relevant but were not seen at the time.

187. Institutions

There are many themes concerned with reactions to arriving at or being in an institution, whether a school, hospital, elderly persons' home or prison (whether as a client or member of staff). They are best tailored to particular needs and institutions. The examples below can be used with clients or staff:

(a) Experiences of first day or first impressions there.
(b) Story of how you came to be there, or in trouble. Can be taken on many levels.
(c) Main concerns, personal or institutional.
(d) How you see yourself, how others see you and how you would like to be seen.
(e) Your institution with yourself in it.
(f) Fold paper in half. Draw your life inside on one half, outside on the other half, and compare.
(g) Your professional self/role. See also (d) above.
(h) Your professional/client relationships (for staff).
(i) A 'rock-bottom' experience and present situation. This focuses on feelings of powerlessness and loss of control.
(j) Situations and feelings which lead up to particular crises, e.g. binge drinking, criminal offence, overdose, etc.
(k) Your goals in your particular institution.
(l) When leaving: feelings about leaving and what your experience here has meant to you.
(m) What your institution does for you; what it does not do for you.
(n) Portrait (realistic or abstract) of facilitator, therapist, teacher. This brings out feelings towards her/him and towards institution.
(o) Feelings about approaching festivals (which may reinforce feelings of isolation, frustration, etc.).
(p) Comic strip of what you would do if you could leave the institution for a few days.
(q) Map of 'organisational geography', e.g. icebergs, sharks, dangerous currents, islands of safety, sheltered harbours, etc. (These metaphors relate to the situation rather than describe particular people.)

(r) Professional issues: use art materials to look at issues such as work conflicts, working with clients, appraisal, professional development, etc. (for details, see Campbell 1993).

(s) Group creates artwork representing what is wrong with their institution, then tries to transform it visually.

References

Campbell, J. (1993) *Creative Art in Groupwork*, Bicester: Speechmark.

Donnelly, M. (1983) 'The origins of pictorial narrative and its potential in adult psychiatry', unpublished research diploma thesis, Department of Art Therapy, Gloucester Rouse, Southmead Hospital, Bristol.

Liebmann, M. (1990) '"It just happened": looking at crime events', in M. Liebmann (ed.) *Art Therapy in Practice*, London: Jessica Kingsley Publishers.

F   Family relationships

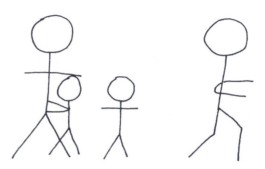

Ideas about families have undergone a major shift during the last 20 years. The concept of a family of two married adults with two children as the norm has given way to a broader view of family including single-parent families, 'reconstituted' families, gay and lesbian couples with children, grandparent-led families, and the wider networks of many cultures now living in the UK. So family can include all of these and any group living together in close proximity or with close ties.

Many ideas in other sections can be adapted to 'family' use. The ones given here are specific to families. They are in two sections:

- Perceptions of family – individual exercises about family relationships.
- Families in action – group activities for families to examine the way they relate to each other in the present.

Perceptions of family

Perceptions of family themes examine how we perceive our relationships with our families. Most people have strong feelings about their families, so sensitivity will be needed in introducing these. It is important to allow plenty of time for discussion. Some of these themes can be particularly

difficult for certain groups of people, e.g. the recently bereaved or those
who have been orphans.

188. Family Portraits

Portraits can be either realistic or use any of the devices in Section I, nos.
272, 273, 286, 287. One method is to describe, as if to a stranger on a train,
the others in your family and how to recognise them. These can then be
portrayed in paint or clay. Variations:

(a) Self-portrait using same method.
(b) Members of family as animals or objects (see no. 286).
(c) Simply draw your family.
(d) Carry on dialogue between family members in painting.
(e) Cut out pictures which remind you of your family.
(f) Cut out coloured paper shapes to represent members of your family.

189. Kinetic Family Drawings

Draw your family with all the members doing something, or the family as a
whole doing something or going somewhere, or a scene from family life.
Variations:

(a) Specify more closely, e.g. a day out with family, etc.
(b) The role you play in your family.
(c) Given a house plan (or plans, if the family is split or reconstituted), put
    in family members and describe the activities.

190. Family Sculpture of Relationships

Represent your family relationships by modelling each member in a characteristic position in relation to others. This can be done with clay or using
a live group of people. Variations:

(a) Sociogram illustrating self in relation to family using size of circle and
    distance apart to signify importance and emotional distance.
(b) Family mobile: 3-D sociogram using coat-hanger, cardboard and
    string.
(c) Pictures of different family relationships.

191. Family Trees

Draw a genogram for your family (this is a family tree with extra information). See books on family therapy for details of genograms, e.g.

Burnham (1986), McGoldrick et al. (1999) or other family therapy books. Add colours and pictures to make it reflect feelings and relationships. Variations:

(a) Family tree: family as a tree with a part assigned to each member, or family members in characteristic positions on branches, according to distance from self. (Imagine going to sleep in a tree and waking to find members of your family or those close to you all saying 'Hello'. Paint their positions – near you perhaps, or even falling out of the tree. Useful way of approaching family issues with children.)
(b) Family tree as above, but add roots and trunk for heritage and journey to present.

192. Inheritance

Fold paper in four and depict in each section:

- what you have inherited
- what you would have liked to inherit
- what you most disliked inheriting
- what you would like your children to inherit.

Variations:

(a) Family past, present and as you would like it to be.
(b) Strengths and weaknesses received from each parent.

193. Family Comparisons

Select a relevant theme from Section E (Self-perceptions) and after doing it for yourself, repeat for others in your family: e.g. parent(s), carer(s), partner, children, etc. Are there any similarities?

194. Childhood Memories

Do a family sculpture (see no. 190) representing a time during your childhood. Memories of childhood often remind people of long-forgotten hurts, which can be upsetting. It is important to be aware of this and allow time for their expression. Variations:

(a) Imaginative journey to childhood to bring back memories (see also no. 147).

(b) Paint yourself now, the things you like, body image, occupations, etc. Then do the same for some point in your childhood.
(c) Make dolls' houses representing various stages of identification, e.g. grandparents, parents, children's home, etc.

195. Re-enacting Parental Relationships

Split into two groups 'parents' and 'children'. Do various role plays emphasising relationship, e.g. blind walks, rocking, etc. Then 'children' draw pictures for 'parents/carers', who provide the materials; 'parents/carers' play with 'children' or do a picture for them. Discussion on parent/child relationships. Variations:

(a) Draw your parent(s)/carer(s) criticising you (or similar statement according to situation).
(b) Fingerpaint to transactional analysis statements made by facilitator ('parent', 'adult' or 'child' statements, e.g. 'Go to your room', 'I appreciate your opinion', 'Let's play'). For an introduction to transactional analysis, see Harris (1995).
(c) Paint the group as a family, allocating roles.

196. Family Themes

There are any number of themes which can be memories, feelings, discussion about families, for example:

(a) Yourself and one other member of the family.
(b) A memory from your childhood.
(c) You and your parents/carers, etc.
(d) Family events, e.g. weddings, births, deaths, gatherings, etc.
(e) Family celebrations.
(f) Family issues.
(g) What the family needs to let go of.
(h) How family members perceive themselves and how other family members perceive them.
(i) Trust.

197. Bereavement Issues

These need to be handled extremely sensitively and may include:

(a) Sharing and doing pictures around losses.
(b) Collages/pictures around own identity and changes in this.

(c) Sharing resources, both personal and practical.
(d) Expressions of anger and rage.

See also no. 284 Bereavement Balloons.

198. Family Relationships Through Play

Children often find it difficult to articulate their feelings in a direct way, but can enact situations through other means, for example:

(a) Sand play: use sandbox and miniature figures of animals and people to portray situations and tell stories, which may have a bearing on family life.
(b) Paper figures: fold and cut paper dolls and animals, evolving stories about animal and human families as you proceed.
(c) Use playdough (see no. 75 for recipes) to make figures of importance to the child, and see what they do and say.
(d) Use a family of dolls to describe situations and feelings.

Families in action

These ideas are for families or couples to explore their actual relationships; for instance, in family therapy sessions. Some of these exercises can enable quiet family members to make an equal contribution. However, they may thus uncover truths that some family members find difficult to accept. Support may be needed to help these families come to terms with what is revealed and, if appropriate, to find new ways of relating to each other.

199. Realistic Family Portraits

Each person draws a picture of the family, making full figures (rather than stick figures) of all individuals, including oneself.

200. Abstract Family or Marital Relationships

Each person draws at the same time, on separate sheets of paper, an abstract or symbolic picture of the family or marital relationship.

201. Couple Relationships

There are several ways of looking at couple relationships, such as:

(a) Both partners make images of the good and bad aspects of their relationship, then discuss these.

(b) Partners each make an image showing how they think the other partner views the relationship.
(c) Focus on a particular aspect.
(d) Divide a piece of paper into three. Each partner does an image about 'how I am feeling' in one of the spaces. The third section is for them to create something together.

202. Emotional Portraits

Partners draw emotional portraits of each other. They then swap pictures and change their portraits as they would like them to be.

Variation: make large realistic self-portraits, give to partner to change as wished.

203. Present Situation

All members of the family draw pictures of the situation now, and as they would like to see it. Looking at the differences can help families set their own goals for change.

Variation: A frustrating moment and a pleasant surprise from the past week.

204. Important Things

Families draw at home those things most important to them and bring their drawing(s) along to the next session for discussion.

205. Shared Experience

Each member of the family draws a picture of her/himself and what she/he was doing at the weekend. These are compared and discussed. Variations:

(a) Other scenes from family life.
(b) See no. 189, Kinetic Family Drawings.
(c) Use any theme from Perceptions of Family section and compare pictures.

206. Problems and Problem Solving

Each member of the family depicts the prevalent problem in their family and how it has affected their life as an individual, e.g. alcohol, criminal offences, mental illness, overdoses, disability, unemployment, etc.

Variation: If there is a particular problem facing a family, or one member of it, each person depicts how they view the problem, their needs and their feelings about it. The different views are then discussed and if possible a course of action clarified.

207. Imagined and Real

Family members reflect (with pictures) on how they imagined relationships were going to be, and how they are in reality.

208. Anger

Members of the family each draw a picture related to their anger. They are then asked to give it to another member of the family.

209. Parents and Children

Children draw pictures of themselves when younger. Parents/carers draw pictures of themselves at ages similar to one of their children. This may bring out similar roles, problems, projections, identifications, etc.

210. Role Reversal

See no. 238, Power Roles, with child bossing parent/carer.

211. Family Circumstances

Each member of the family does a drawing or collage to show the good and bad things about their family circumstances, e.g. being part of a single-parent family; being part of a large/small family, etc.

212. Grandparents' Influence

This is in two parts:

(a) Each member of family draws symbolic picture of family (see no. 200).
(b) Divide paper in half. On one side draw symbolic picture of maternal grandparents' family. On the other side draw the paternal grand-parents' family. After completion, mark which of the two more nearly resembles the picture done in (a).

This exercise can be useful in tracing unconscious heritage from previous generations.

213. Family Sculpture in Action

See no. 190, Family Sculpture of Relationships, but in the present, using family members.

214. Family Drawing or Painting

The family members draw or paint together on one large sheet of paper. They then discuss the family dynamics. Variations:

(a) Family first decides what painting will be about.
(b) Joint construction project, using any materials.
(c) Picture of family in their home.
(d) Picture of everyone doing something.
(e) Create a safe environment for everyone in the family.
(f) Make a messy picture, then transform it into something beautiful.

215. Sharing Resources

A family is given a set of materials to create a family sculpture. The materials can include various things such as a cardboard base, scissors, glue, oil pastels and sheets of stiff paper of different colours, but there should be fewer sheets of paper than members of the family, so that they have to decide how to allocate resources (e.g. four sheets for family of five).

216. Adding to Pictures

Each member of the family has a choice of materials and is allotted a space in the room. Each does her/his own picture for a few minutes, then everyone is free to move around and draw on other people's paper.

Variation: family members add qualities they feel others have/should have.

217. Teams

Each member of the family chooses a different colour crayon or marker. Family divides into two teams and each team produces a picture by the members taking turns, in silence. This may pick up 'family alliances' and the way they work.

218. Art Evaluation Session

This is a series developed by art therapists working in family and marital therapy. Spend about ten minutes on each task, followed by 10 to 15 minutes' discussion. This series is based on work by Kwiatkowska (1978).

(a) Realistic family portrait, see no. 199.
(b) Abstract family or marital relationship, see no. 200.
(c) Joint scribble, see no. 225(g).
(d) Self-portrait given to partner, see no. 202.
(e) Individual pictures, no subject given.

219. Other Pair or Group Activities

Use any of the pair or group activities in Sections G, H and I, as appropriate. These may be revealing, but also a source of shared enjoyable activity which can be important for families.

References

Couple and family techniques

Arrington, D. B. (2001) *Home Is Where the Art Is: An Art Therapy Approach to Family Therapy*, Springfield, IL: C.C. Thomas.
Kwiatkowska, H. (1978) *Family Therapy and Evaluation Through Art*, Springfield, IL: C.C. Thomas.
Landgarten, H. (1987) *Family Art Psychotherapy: A Clinical Guide and Casebook*, New York: Brunner/Mazel.
Linesch, D. (1997) *Art Therapy with Families in Crisis: Overcoming Resistance Through Nonverbal Expression*, New York: Brunner/Mazel.
Linesch, D. (2000) *Celebrating Family Milestones: By Making Art Together*, Toronto: Firefly Books.
Proulx, L. (2003) *Strengthening Emotional Ties through Parent–Child-Dyad Art Therapy*, London: Jessica Kingsley Publishers.
Wadeson, H. (1980) *Art Psychotherapy*, Chichester: Wiley.

Family therapy and genograms

Burnham, J. (1986) *Family Therapy*, London: Tavistock.
McGoldrick, M., Gerson, R. and Shellenburger, S. (1999) *Genograms: Assessment and Intervention*, 2nd edn, New York: Norton.

Other

Harris, T. A. (1995) *I'm O.K. – You're O.K.*, London: Arrow Books.

G Working in pairs

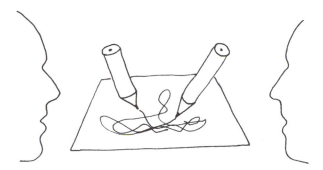

This section includes exercises and activities requiring pairs. Many of these are about the relationship between the pair. There are several variations in the 'ground rules' which affect the interaction. For most of them it is best to work in silence, letting the painting/drawing, etc. take the place of words.

220. Drawing and Painting in Pairs

Paint in pairs on the same piece of paper. If having no other rules is too daunting, try the effect of some different rules, for example:

(a) One person draw curves, the other straight lines.
(b) Each person sticks to a certain colour or colours.
(c) Each mirrors what the other draws, simultaneously.

221. Conversations

Choose a colour that expresses an aspect of yourself and silently pair up with someone who has a different colour. Then have a conversation in paint or crayons on the same paper, each using one colour, one at a time, keeping to your own line. Variations:

(a) Use colours and shapes, any sort of marks, and reply to them.
(b) Stipulate kind of conversation, e.g. getting angry.
(c) One person at a time, while other watches, then other starts where first person left off.
(d) Both work simultaneously taking own lines for a walk.
(e) Following each other.
(f) Exchange colours after a while.
(g) Develop into shared drawing.
(h) Use opposite hand from usual one.
(i) 'Dinner table': with pairs on opposite sides of a long sheet of paper, start conversation with opposite person, then develop conversation with neighbours on either side.

222. Pencil and Paper Friendliness

These are simple exercises to explore the effect of different kinds of behaviour on relationships. In each one, partners have a pencil each (or crayons of different colours) and one sheet of paper between them. The instructions in each case should be given on slips of paper so that partners do not know what the other person's instructions are. If A and B are the partners, here are some possibilities:

(a) *A*: Move around, with the pencil staying on the paper, but try to get away from B.
      B: Try to stay as close to A's pencil/crayon as possible.
(b) *A*: Stay still.
      B: Do everything you can to get A to move their pencil/crayon.
(c) *A*: Don't let B use the paper (but remind them of ground rules).
      B: Use the paper to make as much mess as you can.
(d) *A*: Doodle and do your own thing.
      B: Copy whatever A does.
(e) *A*: Act as if the paper is all yours.
      B: Act as if the paper is all yours.
(f) *A*: Resist using the paper.
      B: Try to persuade A to draw.
(g) *A*: Defend your half of the paper.
      B: Make sure you use the whole page.
(h) *A*: Get in B's way.
      B: Do your own thing.

Many more can be devised.

223. Painting with an Observer

One member of a pair says what comes to mind as she/he watches another paint. The painter responds as she/he sees fit.

Variation: Watcher mirrors artist's rhythm and way of working. Can also have third person observing both. Rotate roles.

224. Sharing Space

Start by taking turns on the same paper, then continue by drawing simultaneously. Look at the way you have structured the space. Variations:

(a) Select three colours between you and draw the experience of your relationship, especially how you are sharing the space.
(b) Exchange colours after a while.
(c) Use collage methods, each person has different colour sticky paper to make pattern on large sheet in common.

225. Joint Pictures

Do a picture with a partner, preferably in silence. Respond to each other's communications and maintain the relationship while painting. Good for meeting new people and for the risk taking involved. Variations:

(a) Simply paint in pairs in silence.
(b) Draw/paint with talking about the task, to compare with (a).
(c) Create an environment for both to exist in.
(d) Start with own colour and eyes closed for two minutes, then work together on result.
(e) Agree on a theme beforehand.
(f) Work with partner to produce a picture which is a cohesive whole.
(g) Each partner makes own scribble, with eyes closed. Then both make associations with results and decide on one scribble to develop into a picture. When the picture is complete, make up a story about it.
(h) Make clay pieces together.

226. Squiggles (based on the work of Winnicott 1971[1982])

Do a squiggle, then swap with partner, who tries to make an image out of it. Good for warming up or for getting imagination going when a group is stuck or flagging. Variations:

(a) Reflect on any assumptions made in giving the squiggle or receiving the completed one.

(b) Paint a symbol or representation of a current moment or concern. Swap silently with partner and continue on his/hers, not obliterating anything. Discuss interplay of interpretations and fantasy.

(c) Draw something and then exchange to work on partner's. Can be theme oriented or anything that comes to mind.

227. Introduction Interviews

Interview partner and then make picture to show something about partner's life and concerns.

228. Dialogue

Paint something to express a current feeling or concern. Partner paints something in response. Reverse roles and repeat. Variations:

(a) Partners each work on own part of picture simultaneously, then swap to respond.

(b) Draw problem on left, exchange, partner draws solution on right.

(c) First person draws situation of concern and describes it. Second person works on drawing to make improvements to situation and describes these. Then both discuss and add further improvements. Then reverse roles.

(d) Dangerous journey. One person draws a path and a hazard, other person draws solution.

229. Sequential Drawings

First person draws characters, second person writes dialogue, etc., to create continuous story.

Variation: First and second persons take turns drawing to create story, no written dialogue.

230. Portraits

Draw a self-portrait and a portrait of your partner. This results in four portraits altogether, which are then shared and discussed. Variations:

(a) Portrait of partner in colours and shapes.

(b) Draw self-portrait, then exchange with partner for further additions. Draw portrait of partner and exchange for additions.

(c) Draw your partner, looking when not drawing.

(d) After drawing portraits, interview your partner.

(e) Pay special attention to details such as buttons, belts, etc.
(f) Use collage to get different effects.

231. First Impressions

Similar to Portraits (no. 230). Relax and look at each other. On a shared piece of paper, take turns to draw anything to which eyes are attracted in partner's face, without lifting crayon from paper. Discuss results when finished. Variations:

(a) On shared paper, take turns to put down first impressions, thoughts or feelings, using abstract means.
(b) Paint impressions of partner using one shape and one colour.
(c) Paint portrait of partner's face, giving an impression of the sort of person.
(d) Paint pictures of the sort of person you are for your partner and the sort of person she/he is for you.
(e) Make portraits of each other and below them write affirmative statements about partner.

232. Masks

Make a mask (or use a prepared blank mask) and paint on it an impression of your partner while she/he is wearing it. Variations:

(a) Make and paint a mask, or several masks. Work with partner, trying on masks.
(b) See also Masks (no. 134). Do these in pairs.
(c) Make masks for each other of the 'front(s)' the other person wears. (It is sometimes easier for others to be aware of our 'fronts' than we are ourselves.)
(d) Use collage materials or media images cut from magazines.
(e) Work in pairs to do plaster of Paris masks from plaster bandages (see no. 134 (g)).

233. Face Painting

Similar to Masks, but using the 'real thing'! In pairs, paint your partner's face with your impression of what sort of person she/he is.
   Variation: Using your partner's face as a canvas, paint an abstract design or expressive mask, taking your time.

234. Silhouettes

Using a piece of paper and a lamp, work in pairs to draw round each other's shadows. Draw in details on partner's silhouette. Variations:

(a) Move about to notice different shadows in different positions.
(b) Simply fill in own silhouette in black.
(c) With children, if the whole room is darkened, those waiting for their turn can work on clay or something else, enjoying and coming to terms with the 'scary' atmosphere.

235. Relationships

Use any combination of warm-up games, followed by both partners painting on a chosen personal theme from Section E (Self-perceptions). The resulting paintings are then shared. Finally, draw or paint the relationship you have built up with your partner, either individually or together.

236. Joint Project

Undertake a joint activity with your partner, e.g. drawing, painting, collage, sculpture, building something. Conversation encouraged.
    Variation: jointly make object from junk materials, no speaking.

237. Joint Control

Two people hold the same pencil and draw with it, without talking, for five minutes. Then talk about the experience and any parallel situations in other parts of your life.

238. Power Roles

One person tells the other which art materials to use, how to use them and what to paint/draw, etc. Reverse roles. Discuss experience. This will bring up issues of power, control and authority. Particularly useful in providing situation in which roles can be reversed from normal ones, e.g. child bosses parent or teacher.

239. Conflicts

Draw or paint a conflict in your life (external or internal). Ask your partner to guess what is going on. Reflect on what is said.
    Variation: after doing the picture, share with a partner. Then swap pictures. Each person then looks at their partner's picture and does another

picture, using the same colours and shapes but arranged differently, in a way that might suggest a solution. Partners share with each other and reflect on how far the new picture suggests a way forward or a different way of viewing the conflict.

References

Winnicott, D. W. (1971) *Playing and Reality*, London: Taylor and Francis Books Ltd; London: Tavistock Publications, 1971; London: Routledge, 1982.

H   Group paintings

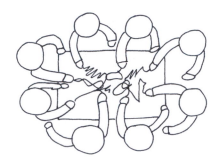

All the items in this section are group paintings in which several people contribute jointly to one piece of paper or one finished product. The differences between group paintings lie in the ground rules set out. Each of the ideas below has selected a different set of these rules, which then influences what happens. (The type of group, setting, environment, etc. also influences what happens, of course. See Part I, Chapter 2.) As well as showing individuals' perceptions, group paintings often reveal very power-fully (and sometimes painfully) some of the group dynamics operating. Some useful questions may be asked about group interaction:

- How does the art form get started?
- Who takes the initiative?
- Whose suggestions are used? Ignored?
- Do people take turns, form teams or work simultaneously?
- Is anyone left out?
- Where is each person's work situated and how much space is used?
- Do people add to others' work?
- Who is the leader or most active participant?
- What influence do different kinds of boundary have?
- Is group painting an enjoyable or a threatening experience?

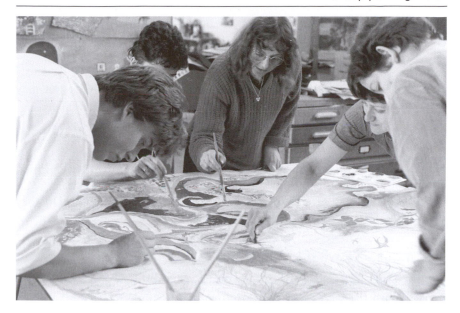

Figure H.1   Group painting in process — staff group at psychiatric hospital
Source: Photograph by John Ford

Not all of the questions on the previous page are relevant or beneficial to every situation. It depends on how much exploration is seen as valuable. Figure H.1 shows a staff group at a psychiatric hospital at work on a group painting.

240. Group Painting with Minimal Instructions

At its most basic, a group is simply presented with a huge sheet of paper (on floor or tables) and asked to work as a group on one large picture with no specified theme. Many of the questions at the beginning of this section will be relevant to the discussion. Variations which may be used to add the desired amount of structure to this situation include:

(a) Each person selects one colour and keeps it, or changes it later if desired, or negotiates with others for colours to mix with the first one.
(b) All start painting at same time.
(c) Work in pairs or teams.
(d) Work cooperatively.
(e) Theme can be decided by group or arrived at in the course of the painting.
(f) All start in centre of paper, or all start at edge of paper.
(g) Take turns for two minutes each, then 'free for all'.

(h) Use fingers and hands.
(i) Use rollers and sponges
(j) Move round the paper.
(k) Choose whether to do the painting in silence or with talking.
(l) Tape the sheet of paper to a wall. This will increase visibility but may make the top less accessible (see Figure H.1).

241. Cooperative Painting

Huge group painting on unspecified theme, but working in with each other, linking own part to neighbour's part. Build up shared experience.

Variation: discuss effects of framework and rules (see above). Do they help or hinder growth of group experience?

242. A Cohesive Whole

Each person draws a picture for ten minutes on an individual piece of paper. When the pieces of paper are turned over, they have numbers and letters on, for example: 1A, 1B, 3C, 3D, etc. These are sellotaped in a grid:

1A   1B 1C 1D
2A   . . .
3A   . . . etc.

The complete set is turned over once more and the group has to make the picture into a cohesive whole, without talking.

Variations:

(a) On a large piece of paper, each person makes a spontaneous scribble. The group then makes a cohesive whole out of these.
(b) A large piece of paper is cut into irregular pieces. Members of the group work on these pieces and then bring them together.

243. Moving On

Everyone starts around a huge piece of paper, does some painting or drawing, and then moves on one place.

244. Picking Out Images

The group covers the paper with spontaneous colours and shapes. Then the paper is passed around and members pick out images they see and emphasise them by drawing them in.

Variations: talk about one of the shapes (liked or disliked) in the first person.

245. Own Territories

Members draw out their own territories, mark them with their names and put in something of themselves. Then everyone is free to put anything else into other people's territorial spaces. Discussion can include who gave what to whom, etc. Variations:

(a) Give other people something you think they need.
(b) Allow 10 to 15 minutes for initial claiming of areas. Finish by returning to own area to make final changes or additions.
(c) After working on initial territories containing selves, link up with other territories.

246. Group Mandala

On a big sheet of paper, draw a large circle and divide it into sectors like pieces of cake, according to the number of people in the group. Individuals can decide whether they wish to remain in their own territories, portraying anything they wish, or whether they also want to enter other people's spaces. Individuals also decide whether their boundaries are to be firm or blended in with those of neighbours on either side. Discussion can look at how people's decisions affected the whole painting and the interactions between people. Variations:

(a) Divide large circle into smaller concentric rings, one for each person.
(b) Choose a theme for whole group, e.g. day and night.

247. Individual Starting Points

Each person takes one colour and with eyes closed takes a line for a walk. After a few minutes, everyone opens their eyes and develops their own spaces with all colours, merging with others at the boundaries. Variations:

(a) The initial stage can involve some moving around the paper.
(b) The later stages can include working on the picture as a whole.
(c) Discussion can be in the whole group, or include conversations with neighbours on the paper.
(d) 'Back to childhood' version: choose an age between 5 and 18 before starting with own line and space.

248. Group Stories

Each person begins to paint a story somewhere on the paper, or from own space. As everyone expands and comes across other people's stories, allow these individual stories to develop and include others' aspects. Move around the paper. Variations:

(a) Move around the paper in turn to add to each story, until arriving back at your own.
(b) Depict common story or event around the paper.
(c) Start with drawing of 'where you feel you are' at edge of paper. Then move on to continue others' stories.

249. Fairy Story in Time Sequence

Each person draws his/her own fairy story in time sequence, on a long sheet of paper (initial agreement on top, bottom, beginning and end of paper). Anyone can start anywhere. No talking. Variations:

(a) Everyone writes a short story, poem or some words about the finished painting or the process of doing it. Those who wish then read theirs out to the group.
(b) Further poems, stories or paintings inspired by the group painting.

250. One-word-at-a-time Story

Each person says a word in turn, to make up a story, which is written down. This story is then illustrated either by individual paintings or by a group painting. Variations:

(a) Paint a story, using people's images to make the story grow.
(b) Pass a painting around, telling a story as you add to it.

251. One-at-a-time Group Drawing

On a large piece of paper, one person starts, others watching. Then the next continues, and so on. Variations:

(a) Start with a story, next person continues.
(b) Make marks in response to what has gone before.
(c) Use only dots, straight lines or curves, first black and white, later perhaps using colours.
(d) Have a fixed number of turns, or stop by common consent.
(e) Pass paper round if small.
(f) Project into picture (if abstract) and draw fantasies of what is seen.
(g) Take turns with drawing something about yourself. Finally, add to whole if wished.
(h) Introductions: name plus picture of self, on sheet on wall.

(i)   Theme murals: after discussion of theme, each person goes to mural in turn and draws.
(j)   Use paints and blocks of colour rather than lines.
(k)   Clay: pass round a lump of clay. Each person does something quickly and then passes it on. Discuss feelings associated with changes.
(l)   Take turns to build a 3-D structure.

252. Group Murals on Themes

These are murals – on large sheets of paper pinned to the wall or on blackboards – on specified themes that are chosen by the facilitator or the group, or arrived at by discussion or by calling out ideas. They can be worked on by one person at a time or by the whole group simultaneously (provided the group is not too large). Examples of themes:

(a)   Facets of life at any particular centre, institution, etc.
(b)   Group events, e.g. outing, picnic, party, etc.
(c)   Feelings about a common experience to group.
(d)   Fantasy themes such as travel, life under the sea, life in outer space, animals, etc.
(e)   Four seasons.
(f)   Abstract design.
(g)   Messages for others, e.g. next group.
(h)   Earth, air, fire, water: divide group members into these four elements (or people choose). Then paint from four corners in the different styles, or all paint anywhere in their element's style.

253. Wall Newspaper/Graffiti Wall

Provide a large sheet of paper on the wall, plus felt-tip pens (tied on with string!). Anyone can write or draw anything at any time. Good for letting off steam and expressing ideas anonymously (e.g. at a conference).

254. Graffiti Anger Wall

Tape a large sheet of paper to the wall, preferably outside, or cover the rest of the wall and the floor with polythene sheeting or old sheets (warn group members about the dangers of slipping on these). Group members write or draw everything that makes them feel angry. Use post-it notes if group is not able to work together on this. When everything is on the wall, ask the group to make clay and paint balls and throw them at the wall.
    Firm ground rules are needed: all stay behind a demarcated line, aim at the paper, no damage to people or property apart from the wall. People can

be encouraged to shout their anger as well. Good for adolescents, but needs a lot of care. Allow plenty of time to discuss afterwards.

255. Combined Anger Symptoms

Based on no. 158, Anger. Starting with an outline of a person on a large sheet of paper, group members take turns to add physical symptoms of anger; either their own or those they have noticed in others. The person ends up looking very angry indeed.

256. How We See Each Other

Tape a very large piece of paper on the wall and divide it into boxes, each with a figure in it and a title at the top. These titles reflect the group and the projections often made about them and by them; for example, when working with young people:

- What young people think of young people.
- What young people think of parents/teachers/police, etc.
- What young people think parents/teachers/police think of young people.

Ask the young people to write and draw their thoughts in each box, add clothes to the figure, etc. When the boxes are full, discuss their content and the whole process.

257. Paradox Wall

Tape a large sheet of paper on the wall and divide it in half down the middle. Invite group members to contribute opposite pairs, e.g. love/hate. Then participants write and draw their loves and hates in the two halves (but no names of particular people). This exercise draws out positive as well as negative sides of life and relationships. These can then be discussed. Sometimes people hate things that turn out to be part of themselves as well.

   Variation: use other pairs of opposites, e.g. messages from parents to keep/reject.

258. Solidarity

Sometimes oppressed minorities can find it useful to celebrate their common bonds and their positive contributions by drawing or painting murals depicting their experiences of these. There may be political issues involved, which can generate heated arguments. Examples of themes:

(a) Minority ethnic festivals and music.
(b) Women's contributions to humanity.
(c) Disability issues.
(d) Symbols of peace.
(e) Murals of local activities in the surrounding community.
(f) Development issues.
(g) Problems faced by marginalised groups, e.g. homeless people, ex-prisoners, people with mental health problems, etc.

259. Celebrating Diversity

Group painting/collage of aspects of diversity – culture, heritage, gender, group identity – either by all joining in on the same sheet of paper or by contributing individual panels to the whole.

260. Building Islands and Worlds

The group uses a collection of junk materials, paint, collage, crayons, etc. to build an island or world for the group to live on. Variations:

(a) If several small groups are doing this, they can later visit other islands to compare with their own.
(b) Instead of an island, build a house, park, school, community centre, town, city, world or 'group environment'.
(c) Use crayons or paint instead of junk materials.
(d) Specify more conditions, e.g. town on particular occasion, stranded on an island, meeting survival needs, aerial view of village with participants developing own areas and working or living communally.
(e) Draw individual islands on mural. Then choose someone else's island to visit and devise means of getting there. If appropriate, discuss reasons for choice.
(f) Draw individual towns in corners of large sheet of paper. Then make a road to someone else's town (best with groups of four).
(g) Create fantasy community on mural paper with markers or crayons.
(h) Create own house and then make neighbourhood.
(i) Use clay to make clay 'world'.
(j) Create individual clay trees and make a forest on a large board. If outside, also add sticks, leaves and stones.
(k) Individual self boxes (see no. 128), then create an environment for them.
(l) Use collage to make circular 'world'.
(m) Worlds in boxes.

(n) Make full-length self-portrait and put in most suitable place for self. Group discusses and perhaps changes, then creates suitable environment for the self-portraits.

(o) If several groups are involved, final discussion can compare cities or worlds, or evolve criteria for evaluating them.

(p) Picture or sculpture of the group.

261. Group Collage

Many of the ideas listed so far can be translated into collage by using magazines and ready-made images instead of paints or crayons, e.g. using collage for a themed mural, making a world, etc.

Variation (good for children): each child is given total control of at least one piece of equipment (e.g. scissors), which only she/he may use.

262. Feelings Collage

Cut out pictures which clearly express emotion, and paste into a collage. Write what each character might be saying.

Variation: group members can mime or act the feelings expressed.

263. Creating Change

Group painting of what is wrong with an institution or organisation. Then the group transforms the picture visually to envisage positive changes.

Variation: junk sculpture of situation. Then transform to how like it to be. (Junk sculpture can be a good metaphor for building something good out of rubbish or a bad situation.)

264. Contributions

The following are all ideas for group paintings which consist of individual contributions from group members. They are particularly suitable for groups which would not be able to work together in a less structured way.

(a) Assembly of individual panels (previously prepared to fit together) on given themes, in crayon, paint or collage.

(b) Each person assigned a fixed space on a given project.

(c) Jigsaw: cut blank group shape into smaller shapes. Each member fills in one shape, then the larger shape is reassembled.

(d) A large piece of paper is divided into sections meeting at a central circle. Different shapes are assigned to each member, e.g. triangles, squares, stars, etc., with instructions to work towards and enter the centre.

(e) In a group, draw a tree – then everyone puts different things underneath.

(f) Draw a house, then different people put in different rooms and activities.

(g) Four people can use four sides of box to do individual contributions on any theme.

(h) Hand tracings of all members of the group on a large piece of paper. This can be achieved either by everyone taking turns to draw round their hands on the same piece of paper, or by each person doing their own and then cutting it out and sticking it on the group paper.

(i) Discuss how individual contributions are to be fitted together.

265. Moving Closer

For an ongoing group, if working on co-operative projects is difficult, devise stages in moving closer:

(a) Work in allotted space on large paper, physically distant from each other.

(b) Reduce allotted space to increase physical proximity.

(c) Unify individual parts to make a cohesive whole.

(d) All work on one small project, without allotting spaces.

266. Group Sculptures

The group works together on one piece of clay, with no set theme, or to produce a joint sculpture. Variations:

(a) Use a layer of clay in same way as group painting (rather clay consuming).

(b) Use other 3-D materials such as wood offcuts or junk materials.

(c) Good option for working with children: each child has total control of at least one piece of junk, clay, plasticine, etc., which only she/he can use to produce co-operative group sculpture.

(d) Everyone does a part of a particular scene (e.g. park, circus) and then makes it into a whole.

(e) Each person uses different colour of plasticine or other materials so that individual contributions can be seen.

(f) Each person has different materials, e.g. coloured paper, tissue paper, cellophane, etc. First person starts, passes on to next to add something, and so on.

267. Overlapping Group Transparency

This is good for a group which has worked together on another project or been together for some time. Each person chooses a different colour of cellophane and uses it to represent her/himself in the group, according to shape, size and position. Using coloured cellophane means that the way the group functions can also be shown, by overlapping the individual shapes.

268. Group Roles

Each person makes a three-dimensional self-image (in clay, plasticine, wood scraps or other junk materials), then moves it about in silence on a large piece of paper or board which acts as a 'world space'. When each person has found his or her 'spot', this is marked by a line drawing. Then the group discusses the various possible roles in a group, e.g. facilitator, disruptor, outsider, intruder, scapegoat, peacemaker, etc.

269. Role Playing

Group painting with people assigned different roles, preferably role reversals from usual behaviour. Finish by doing individual pictures to go back to 'being oneself'. Variations:

(a) Assign pictorial roles, such as 'paint in yellow', 'take up lots of space', etc.
(b) See no. 252 (h) above.

270. Painting to Music

Paint as a group to music, being aware of group and feelings. Variations:

(a) Warm up by moving to music.
(b) Movement exercises, followed by painting, with movements of different qualities, e.g. bold, sweeping, controlled, etc.

271. Individual Response to Group Painting

Group paintings can be powerful experiences. These may be assimilated better if each member of the group does an individual painting in response to the group painting experience. These may be shared if desired.

I Group interactive exercises

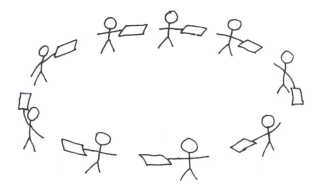

This section includes interactive exercises in which the 'rules for interaction' presuppose a group, although there is often no group end product. Most of the exercises involve comparing one's own perceptions with those of others. Many of them extend ideas from Section E (Self-perceptions) and G (Working in Pairs). Because they take the focus off the individual artwork, these exercises can be a way into using art in a personal way. In some situations they can be experienced as enjoyable games. However they can often also give a new perspective on serious concerns. Particular care is needed if groups include vulnerable people.

272. Portraits

Make quick portraits of everyone else (e.g. 10 portraits in 30 minutes). Sign them and give them to the person drawn. Variations:

(a) Suggest portraits should be funny/in shapes and colours/using textures.
(b) Sketches of others in group walking or doing typical activity (can be matchstick figures).

(c) Clay figures: model the figure of another group member in posture that clearly communicates his/her feeling.
(d) Draw portraits of self using distinctive features; comment on own drawings to group. Group supplies nickname possibly, or guesses who drew portraits.
(e) Draw portrait of partner, then others negotiate to work further on portraits.

273. Portraits by Combined Effort

Each member is the subject in turn and draws a self-portrait. Then other members in turn make the portrait more like the subject.

274. Group Hands

On a large piece of paper, everyone in turn draws round one of their hands, using a different colour crayon. This can be a good way of starting a group and of emphasising the contract of confidentiality with the symbolism of overlapping hands.
   Variation: add messages.

275. Badges and Totems

Paint a badge to describe yourself and pin it on. Then make similar badges for others, describing their main characteristics. Works best when people know each other well, or in a group of people prepared to take risks. Variations:

(a) Put individual badges on group 'totem pole'.
(b) Make large totem pole with cardboard boxes. Members of group decorate with personal symbols.
(c) Coats of arms for yourself and others.

276. Empathy Hats

Explain the meaning of empathy, with examples. Group members make hats from card and other materials, with feelings inside and outside according to whether they show them. These are discussed. Then group members try on each other's hats and talk about how they felt doing this. Useful for children to learn to understand others' feelings. (Be aware of the different cultural issues around head covering and the meanings of hats.)
   Variation: individuals think of a feeling they experience a great deal and make a hat portraying this. Then people swap hats and explore the feelings portrayed in their own experience.

277. Understanding and Recognising Feelings

Therapist/facilitator draws simple faces on cards to show 'happy', 'sad' and 'angry'. Group members demonstrate these to each other. A mirror can be useful to help them see their own expressions. Then group members cut out faces from magazines or collage collections to make group pictures for each of these feelings. A variety of facial colours and backgrounds should be included.

278. Different Points of View

Starting from a problem situation, different members of the group illustrate the situation from a different person's point of view. The pictures are shared and the differences discussed.

279. Cultural Identities (based on no. 133 (h))

If there are members of different cultural groups (this can be taken to mean any groups with different identities), each group can be asked to develop two group images, one of which they think may be perceived as threatening, the other as non-threatening. These can then be tested out with the other groups. (Not suitable if there is a large imbalance of numbers belonging to the different groups.)

280. Group Symbol

The group develops and paints a symbol which is shared by the whole group.
　　Variation: group coat of arms.

281. Masks

Everyone paints a mask, then wears it and takes part in plays involving the mask's character; best done in small groups, say fours. There are many variations and ways of achieving the chosen masks, for example:

(a) Mask of unacceptable side of your personality. Then get together in fours with opposite masks, forming a 'family unit' to do a role play. Imagination and visualisation techniques can be used to get in touch with the unacceptable side (see Section J).
(b) One person talks about his/her mask and another person acts the role.
(c) Everyone brings an object to the group. Then each person does a mime using all the objects and evolves a 'character' which is then painted on his/her mask. The masks are then used in a play.

(d) Use paperbags and paint to make characters which come alive, and act plays with them (good for children).
(e) Carnival of masks.

282. Gifts

Make, draw or paint gifts you would like to give to each person in the group, and then give them. This can also be done on a large blackboard. Discussion will explore feelings around giving and receiving and possibly around parting with the gifts. Variations:

(a) To end a group, a 'goodbye' gift to take away.
(b) Can be geared to festivals, e.g. Chanucah, Christmas, Diwali, Easter, Id, etc.
(c) Stipulate kind of gift – concrete, abstract, etc.
(d) Can have particular purpose, e.g. to help attain a short-term goal.
(e) Precious objects.
(f) Positive qualities.
(g) Can be repeated at intervals; see if gifts become more relevant.
(h) Make or draw any object, then give it to someone in the group.
(i) On a large piece of paper, everyone draws a box, basket or bag to receive their presents. Then everyone moves round and paints or draws a gift for others – including themselves. After group exchange and discussion (people may want to ask why someone has given them a certain gift), if the exercise is at the end of a group, members cut out their basket to take away with them.
(j) Everyone combines to make something for a person who is leaving/has left. This may include things symbolising what they meant to you, or things you associate with them, or things you wish to give them. People can work together or contribute individual pieces/pictures to be brought together at the end. Meanwhile the person who is leaving can work on a picture to leave to the group.
(k) Wishes and inspirational sayings can be added to any of the above.

283. Affirmation Posters

Place A4 pieces of paper or card on chairs or a table around the room, each with a group member's name at the top. Everyone moves round, writing or drawing something good (or something they have valued during this group) about that person. Good way to end a weekend workshop or a series of sessions. Variations:

(a) Tape the posters to people's backs (be sensitive to groups where touch is not welcome).

(b) For young children, use larger pieces of paper and handprints to make contributions.

284. Bereavement Balloons

Obtain a helium balloon. On small pieces of paper, members of the group draw or paint an image or message to the individual who has died – something they wish they had told that individual when they were alive. After group discussion of images, tie them to the balloon string, then go outside and release the balloon into the sky as the group watches. Return to the room to discuss the whole ceremony.

285. Shared Feelings

Choose a topic of concern to group members, e.g. a shared problem, situation, etc. Each person draws good and bad things about the particular situation, each thing on a separate small piece of paper. Any shared images are then discussed as a set.

286. Metaphorical Portraits: Individuals

Paint metaphorical portraits of others (and self) in the group (see also no. 138). Sometimes there is only time for a few; sometimes everyone can do a portrait of everyone else. The portraits can be abstract or flowers, animals, buildings, trees, houses, islands, symbols, etc. There are several ways of sharing the results:

(a) Everyone takes turns to explain the portraits they have done.
(b) One person holds up a portrait, others guess who it is; the person who guesses correctly then holds up a portrait, and so on.
(c) When each portrait has been discussed or 'guessed', it is given to the subject as a gift. At the end, everyone has a collection of metaphorical portraits of themselves.

Further variations of this idea:

(d) Self and one other – abstracts. This can be specified to be someone in the group or not in the group. The guessing game can then suggest who the other person is.
(e) Draw an imaginary animal, then see what happens when two animals meet.

287. Metaphorical Portrait: Group

Find a metaphor for the group as a whole and paint it. This can be done separately by each individual, or as a group. Variations:

(a) Draw the group as animals with a background.
(b) Draw yourself as part of the group, using colour, position, form, etc. This can be added to or changed over a period of time.
(c) Combine with no. 286. Portray members of group individually and the group as a whole.

288. Interpretations

The basic idea is to compare group interpretations with what was intended. There are many ways of doing this, for example:

(a) See nos. 286, 287(c) (metaphorical portraits of individuals and group). In discussion, everyone else (apart from artist) comments, makes associations and interpretations. Artist keeps silent.
(b) Everyone paints a picture on a specified theme, e.g. a face, a tree, an animal, a house, an island, a mask, etc. The pictures are collected and shuffled, then held up one by one. The group describes each picture in a way that could describe a person.
(c) Everyone paints their ideas of different emotions, e.g. anger, anxiety, etc. and labels each small picture on the reverse. The pictures are mixed up, then the group picks one out and tries to agree on an interpretation. This is then compared with the original intention.
(d) One person describes a picture, which everyone tries to draw from the instructions. The completed pictures are compared with the original and discussion focuses on the different interpretations people make of information given to them.
(e) For children: each child gives a 'word' to another child to depict in some way. Discussion focuses on how children interpreted a particular word.

289. Interpretations in Action

In groups of three, each person paints a symbol or situation of the present. Swap silently and continue, not obliterating anything. Repeat with third person, then back to original. Discuss interpretations.

290. Diversity Maps

Divide into groups to represent different interests, e.g. different areas of the town, different ethnic groups, different age groups, different family members (e.g. parents, teenagers, young children), etc. Ask each subgroup to draw a mental map between them of something or a place in common to everyone in the whole group, e.g our town, important things in our neighbourhood, future arrangement of resources. When the drawings are finished, compare notes on what is included/left out, size and placement of different elements. This leads on to discussion of priorities for different groups.

Variation: if there are impending changes (e.g. a new community centre), whole group can then work on consensus map of changes that best fit everyone.

291. Conflict Cartoons

Groups of two to five people co-operate to produce a cartoon illustrating a conflict or theme they feel is important. Then each group passes their cartoon to another group for interpretation and consideration of bias, stereotypes, viewpoint offered, etc. (This is based on the fact that cartoons often rely on using stereotypes to communicate their message.)

292. Group Problem Solving

This is similar to no. 228(c). One person does a drawing of a difficult situation and describes it. Then other people in the group make improvements to the drawing and discuss these, until the best possible solution is arrived at.

293. Giving Away Stress

Group members draw individual pictures of a current stressful situation. Then they decide what part of their drawing they could give away to contribute to a group picture or mural. Then the group works on the mural to make it into a cohesive whole.

294. Butterflies

Each person makes two butterflies by folding sheets of paper in half on daubs of paint. Put one aside and then do a monoprint of someone else's on top of your second one. Repeat with more interactions on the same one, as many as wished. Discuss fears of loss of identity in group; the clean butterfly can represent preserved identity.

295. Life-size Individuals and Group

Draw outline around each person (see no. 129), then fill in colours in outlines other than your own. Variations:

(a) Put in characteristics of that person.
(b) Others in group put in hat, clothes, shoes, etc.

296. Round Robin Drawings

Number the papers around the group. Everyone draws for two minutes (this needs timing, preferably by a non-participant), then passes on their paper and continues on the next one for one minute; and so on until everyone receives back the one she/he started with and finishes it off for two minutes. No talking. Discussion focuses on people's feelings about the changes in their pictures. Sometimes useful for a new group, as no one has to take responsibility for a whole picture. Variations:

(a) Start by drawing for longer period, e.g. five minutes.
(b) Finish with longer period, e.g. five minutes.
(c) Do the whole exercise very fast.
(d) Specify starting point is something from own situation.
(e) Specify no obliterations.
(f) Reflect on results and do individual drawing to express feelings.
(g) Add a word each when painting is done.
(h) Close eyes, take a line for a walk, open eyes to do some drawing, then pass on to someone else.
(i) Specify a theme, e.g. 'having fun'.
(j) Start with an abstract symbol.
(k) For children: child starts a drawing and asks next child to add to it according to their instructions, e.g. 'I've drawn a car; I'd like you to put some wheels on it.'
(l) Take turns to contribute to a plant: first person draws a seed, next person the soil, then roots, shoots, stem, leaves, buds, flowers, fruits.

297. Scribble, Tear and Reconstruct

Group members scribble on large piece of paper, then tear it into pieces as a group. Each member takes some pieces to make into something individually.

298. Fill in the Gap

Do a picture and leave something out. Someone else has to guess what. Or leave something for someone else to do.

Variation: use this to remind of last session, group and facilitator fill in gaps for each other or catch each other out if they forget anything.

299. Facilitator Draws

Group members tell facilitator what to draw. This gives group members permission to reveal feelings towards authority (facilitators, teachers, parents, etc.), or allows normally passive members to be more active.

Variation for children: child draws picture line by line, stopping while everyone else copies each line. Only the child in the lead knows what the picture will be. The resulting pictures are then compared.

300. Beautiful and Ugly

First person makes something beautiful and this is continued for several passings on. Then it is turned into something ugly; then made good again. Explore the feelings associated with each process. People with very low esteem have difficulty with this one, as they may feel that all their drawings are ugly anyway. Also, some people simply cannot bear the idea of spoiling something on purpose. Variations:

(a) In groups of four to six, alternate members make beautiful, spoil, remake beautiful, etc. Finally, original artist makes it beautiful to finish. Allow five minutes each part. May be a good idea to repeat with group members taking opposite role to first time.
(b) Two groups do a picture each, swap to spoil, then make good again.
(c) Each person does a second picture, including all the good and bad elements, and tries to make them into a 'whole' picture.
(d) Variation for children: child one draws a shape, child two spoils it by drawing a few lines on it, child three repairs it by including the lines in a new design. Or work in pairs, changing something 'ugly' to something 'beautiful'.

301. Secrets

Everyone draws a secret without saying what it is. Discuss what having a secret means. Swap paintings with another person and do a sketch which is a parody of their secret. Discussion.

302. Big Bag of Worries

Provide or make a large box or bag (a large bin liner or rubbish bag of a darkish opaque colour will do) and put it in an accessible place in the room. Members of the group write, draw or sculpt their worries and post or place them in the bag. The group then discusses what to do with them – destroy them, process them or respond with a picture.

303. Pool of Drawings

Everyone begins drawing anything they like. When they feel like it, they place it in the middle of the circle and continue on someone else's drawing. This carries on until it comes to a natural conclusion.

304. Pool of Colours

Give out pieces of card and ask people to paint them a variety of colours. Then cut them up and put the pieces into a pool in the middle. Everyone chooses some pieces and uses them as a basis for making a picture.

305. Group Additions

Each member names an object, event or feeling and depicts it. Then other members add improvements. Discussion of feelings about the changes that are made.

306. Group Sequential Drawing

Divide a piece of paper into numbered squares, one more than the number of people in the group. In the first square draw the beginning of a story (for three minutes). Pass it on and draw in the second square on the next paper. When everyone gets their own back, the end of the story is put in. Discussion. Variations:

(a) Write very quick synopsis of story.
(b) Cut up sections and reassemble own sections, to see if they have any particular theme.
(c) Specify starting point, e.g. important event, childhood memory, etc.
(d) Captions: when papers are passed on each person writes caption on previous drawing before contributing next drawing. Final square: own drawing plus caption.
(e) One piece of paper only, passed around.
(f) Narrative themes, e.g. 'in prison', 'adrift at sea', 'won the lottery', etc.

307. Animal Consequences

Each person draws the head of an animal, folds paper and passes on. Next person draws body, next one legs. Then each person takes one they have not worked on and talks about it in first person.

Variation: the more conventional one, using people. Each person draws a hat, folds paper, passes on; then face, body, legs, feet, etc.

308. Conversations in Paint (based on no.221(i))

Start with pairs opposite each other along long sheet of paper. One colour each, start conversation with opposite person (different colour), then let conversations develop with neighbours on either side, etc.

309. Situation Diagrams

Everyone draws a sketch or diagram to represent what they think is (or was) going on in a particular situation in which the group was involved. Discuss everyone's diagrams in the group, perhaps classify them. This is described in more detail in Cortazzi and Roote (1975).

Variation: to plan action, draw diagram of situation and consider silently (two minutes) possible actions, then discuss.

310. Sociograms

The group draws diagrams to illustrate graphically community relationships, or relationships between individuals. Variations:

(a) Use 3-D materials such as polystyrene balls, wire, string and paint.
(b) Can be used to present graphically information about the group, e.g. answers to the question 'Who in the group do you know best?'
(c) Can be used to plot number of verbal communications from each person to each other person, to give an 'interaction picture'.

311. Creative Thought Streams

The group starts with a key word in the middle of the paper, e.g. JOB or ANGER, etc. Everyone adds any other words that occur to them in 'thought streams'. Then any word that has cropped up can be taken as a basis for individual painting.

312. Visual Whispers

First person shows second a drawing, then asks him/her to sketch it from memory. Second person shows this to third person, who in turn sketches it from memory. Compare last drawing with first. Discuss the sort of distortions which occur.

313. Newspaper Games

These are co-operative games for small groups (four to seven) which can then compare results with other groups.

(a) Animal shapes: each small group has to tear an animal shape out of newspaper, one turn each, no speaking.
(b) Fashion model: each group makes an outfit for a model from newspapers.
(c) Building a tower: each group builds a self-standing tower, to be judged by height, stability and originality (jury formed by members from each group). Allow one hour.
(d) As (c), but time limit of half an hour and repeat three times:
   • verbal communication allowed
   • no verbal communication
   • single words only.

314. Using Magazine Pictures

Everyone selects a magazine picture they like and these are pinned up. Group writes down qualities of picture chosen, then associations to each picture are shared in group. Variations:

(a) Choose pictures disliked.
(b) Given a few photographs from magazine, small groups think up articles to fit them. A 'reporter' tells the story to the large group.
(c) Pairs choose a magazine photograph that shows two people communicating and perform the conversation they might be having. The group guesses which photograph it is.

315. Trading Skills

The group is divided into two halves and both groups have sheets of paper. One group is given materials, e.g. collage materials, paint, etc. The other group is given equipment, e.g. scissors, glue, brushes, etc. The two groups have to trade with each other to provide a collage/painting, etc. People can work individually, in small groups, or as a whole group. The theme can be chosen to reflect conflict at some level (interpersonal, community, national, international) or left to the group. There are many possibilities in trading, e.g. fair trading, driving a hard bargain, etc. The discussion will include what took place and particular sources of conflict, together with any solutions discovered.

316. Art Arena Games

These are co-operative team games developed by Don Pavey (1979) and described fully in his book. The aim is to create a mural from the contributions of two groups (two to four members in each). Below is a summary of the stages involved in an adapted version by Suzanne Charlton (1984):

(a) Fix a large sheet of paper to a wall for the mural.
(b) Divide into two equal groups.
(c) Choose a theme (e.g. a pattern, sunshine and storm, birds, space exploration, carnival) in which two contrasting ideas have to be combined.
(d) Each group chooses colours and shapes to represent their group.
(e) Members of each group draw and paint their own images on separate sheets of paper and cut them out.
(f) Both groups, working at separate tables, arrange layouts for their designs.
(g) The mural: two people (one member from each group) take turns to transfer a cut-out shape on to the mural until all the shapes have been used.
(h) Everyone makes suggestions on moving shapes around to improve the final result.
(i) Discussion of result and process. Some relevant questions might be:

- Is the result a unified picture or not?
- Was the game enjoyable or stressful?
- Did people co-operate or were there problems?

References

Charlton, S. (1984) 'Art therapy with long-stay residents of psychiatric hospitals', in T. Dalley (ed.) *Art as Therapy*, London: Tavistock.

Cortazzi, D. and Roote, S. (1975) *Illuminative Incident Analysis*, New York: McGraw-Hill.

Pavey, D. (1979) *Art-Based Games*, London: Methuen.

J Guided imagery, visualisations, dreams and meditations

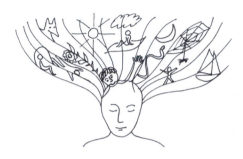

This section includes techniques that aim to get in touch with parts of our consciousness of which we are normally unaware. Some of the images arising from these techniques can be quite powerful and it is important to ensure that people can return to 'normal life' at the end of their experience. The section falls into three parts:

1 Guided imagery and visualisation

    (a) Preparation for visualisations
    (b) Imaginative journeys
    (c) Identifications
    (d) Other ways of stimulating imagery
    (e) Visualising change
    (f) Further reading

2 Dreams, myths and fairy tales
3 Painting as meditation

1. GUIDED IMAGERY AND VISUALISATION

(a) Preparation for visualisations

Before listing some of the themes, let us look at the method itself and the preparation needed to approach it. These themes are sometimes also called guided fantasies, but as they often include a mixture of fantasy and reality, the concepts of imaginative journeys and visualisations seem more accurate.

The basic method is as follows, in its barest outline. Starting with some relaxation exercises, the facilitator tells a story, or describes a scene, concentrating on the sort of details that bring back memories or evoke feelings. After returning from the 'trip', everyone paints an image from it (or, if it is preferred, everyone shares experiences verbally). There are several important points to be borne in mind if you are thinking of using imaginative journeys or visualisations with a group. I have listed these, together with some examples of what can go wrong.

(i) Suitability

They are not appropriate for very disturbed people and work best with groups that can concentrate enough to listen well. Even if there is only one person who is too disturbed, or who cannot concentrate, this may be enough to spoil the experience for others. People also need to be able to relax in order to 'get into' imaginative journeys, so if this is a major problem, the method is not suitable for that group – or some practice with relaxation techniques is needed first.

The main point of many of these journeys and visualisations is to tap unacknowledged parts of the person, and become aware of them, such as hidden needs or strengths. The extent to which this is possible depends on the insight of the people concerned. For people with little insight, the journeys will remain at their face value, but can nevertheless be worthwhile.

(ii) Different levels of experience

They can be used on several different levels: for instance, as story-telling with children or people with learning disabilities, to stimulate their imagination; or as an approach to any theme for adults, to help them feel their way into it. At a deeper level, they can bring up some very powerful images, which can stay with people and sometimes be very upsetting. So care is needed to keep the level light enough for people to cope. If this is done, they can lead to enjoyable and worthwhile experiences.

Example 1

A group of children were asked to imagine themselves going for a walk in the sunshine, along a path that led into a green field. What was in the field? This led to an enjoyable session with many imaginative paintings.

Example 2

A group of professionals was asked to make an imaginative journey to a place they knew and which had special memories, and then do a painting. It was intended to be a positive experience, but the 'special memories' for one person included some acute pain in the resulting painting. This produced a total catharsis which was inappropriate in that particular setting, unexpected for the therapist, and destructive because it was unresolved.

(iii) Levels of relaxation

Some means of relaxation are needed at the beginning, and the level chosen may influence the depth of the subsequent experience. At the lightest level, members of the group just close their eyes so that they can 'see' the images in the story as the facilitator tells it. A useful mid-level of relaxation can be reached by asking people to sit in easychairs, or back to back on the floor, and going through some simple relaxation exercises (close eyes, let go of bags, open hands, feel chair/floor, feet on ground, comfortable). A deeper relaxation is achieved with the group lying on the floor (eyes closed). People are in a state of greater suggestibility in this state. This can be too much for some groups and may be inappropriate in some settings (e.g. short-term groups in which little is known about the participants).

(iv) The journey or visualisation

When people are relaxed, the facilitator tells a story consisting mainly of images, concentrating on the sorts of details that enable people to bring back memories, or to visualise their own version of what is being described. It is important to tell the story or describe the journey slowly to allow people time to select the right memory or see their own details, e.g. of a tree. This process is important and cannot be hurried. Practice is needed to find the right pace.

Example 3

In one group, the leader hurried through the instructions too fast and the group prepared to do paintings without their usual enthusiasm. It turned out that they all felt that they had been whisked through the journey so fast that they had not stayed with any images long enough to be able to paint them. So the facilitator had to start again and go through it more slowly. This time everyone had a personal image to paint and found the session interesting and rewarding.

(v) Coming back

Often in imaginative journeys there is a definite transition point to 'another world', e.g. a door in a garden wall. It is most important to bring people back through that door and back into present time.

Example 4

A group of psychiatric patients was taken on an imaginative journey to outer space, where they landed on a planet and painted, danced or drama-tised what it was like. However, they were never brought back and the group remained disturbed – not only for the rest of the day, but for several weeks in relation to the sessions.

(vi) Painting

At the end of the trip, everyone is asked to paint an image of their trip. This is usually a period of quiet concentration in which people are still 'digesting' their experience. Verbal sharing is probably most usefully left until after this unless there is an obvious need for it.

(vii) Support

It is important to allow time to talk at the end and to have adequate support available in case this is needed. Even well-planned sessions can be unpredictable.

(viii) A first-person account

To conclude, here is a first-person account of a visualisation which resulted in a positive experience:

After a session of movement exercises and a short meditation, we all lay down on the floor and relaxed. Sarah read the 'Wise Person Guide' visual-isation from a book, very slowly and deliberately with long pauses (see no. 318). I was in a forest in springtime, with newly clad beech trees all round. When I approached the fire, the person I met was my favourite adopted aunt, who died several years ago. I asked her whether I was making the right decision (I was considering leaving my job to go on a course). She beamed at me and said: 'You always make wonderful decisions!' She picked up a single new leaf on a twig from the ground and gave it to me. At first I was disappointed with my gift and thought 'Is that all?', but later I realised the freshness of the leaf represented enjoyment of the present moment, which was something I could have at any time and was worth more than any more durable object. Later, I did a painting of myself, my adopted aunt, the fire and the leaf, with a huge beech tree framing them. Doing this painting helped me to absorb the experience, which I found very encouraging.

(b) Imaginative journeys

Below are a few examples of imaginative journeys. In each case, you remain yourself in the journey. Only the 'bare bones' are given, and details need to be filled in to make each one seem more 'real'. This can be done by thinking through the journey beforehand.

317. Magic Carpet Ride

Outdoors on a beautiful spring day . . . sunshine . . . imagine being on a magic carpet, free to travel anywhere without any effort . . . feel yourself floating off the ground . . . go as high as you wish . . . look down . . . remain calm and relaxed . . . go anywhere you want . . . take a few minutes for your journey . . . return . . . savour any special moment.

318. Wise Person Guide

Outdoors on a calm sunny day . . . find self in clearing in wood . . . notice smells and sounds . . . feels very safe . . . path leads up through woods . . . come to a clearing . . . fire in middle . . . on other side of fire is your wise person guide, waiting quietly . . . place log on fire . . . go and sit with wise person. . . what is she/he like? . . . when ready, ask a question . . . listen for answer . . . rest a while, and thank your guide . . . she/he embraces you as you leave and gives you a gift in memory of your meeting . . . back down the path calmly . . . to first clearing.

319. Gifts

You are in a beauty spot by a warm lagoon . . . you dive in, find some underwater rocks . . . there is a cave . . . you swim through . . . find an opening . . . then meet someone who gives you a gift . . . you receive this and return through the cave. Afterwards, paint the person you met and the gift you received.

320. Secret Garden and House

You are walking through some woods . . . find a path . . . follow it . . . come to a gate in a wall . . . go through . . . private/secret garden . . . explore it . . . see a house . . . decide whether to go in or not . . . what is it like? . . . maybe meet someone . . . what happens? . . . and return through gate and path.

321. Secret Cave

Go for a walk . . . come to a meadow . . . sunshine . . . tree . . . flowers . . . look at them, feel and smell them . . . stream . . . boat . . . into a tunnel secret cave . . . what do you find? . . . returning from the cave . . . and so back home.

322. Doorway

Go for a walk . . . find a doorway . . . what is it like? Familiar or unfamiliar? . . . decide to open the door . . . is it hard or easy? . . . open the door and go through . . . what do you find?

323. Mountain View

Pastoral scene . . . mountains . . . climb up . . . describe the journey . . . reach the top . . . look at the view . . . meet special person . . . what sort of conversation do you have? . . . ask that person a question . . . what do you ask? . . . what is the reply? . . . come down from the mountain.

324. Farm

Walking around a farm . . . through fields . . . describe the fields . . . into the farmyard . . . describe the yard and buildings . . . name the different kinds of animal . . . and the farmer . . . come back to the room . . . paint an animal or person from the farm and their surroundings.

325. Magic Shop

Going out for a trip . . . visit a sleepy old village . . . find a shop . . . a magic shop . . . what do you find in it? . . . what do you take back with you? (or a magic junk-shop in a backstreet of a busy town . . .)

326. Boat Journey

Starting out in a boat . . . where does it start from? . . . where is it going? . . . what is the journey like?. . . how does it end? Make up your own story, and then draw or paint it.

327. Shipwrecked on an Island

You are shipwrecked on an island . . . you land . . . what is it like? . . . what do you do first? . . . if you are part of a group, what do you decide to do all

together? . . . how do you get rescued? . . . what do you feel when you
return?

328. Hidden Seed

Visualise a landscape without life . . . imagine a little seed which has
remained hidden for a long time . . . where is it? . . . what might happen if it
was watered and cared for? . . . does the seed grow? . . . what happens to it?

329. Five Senses

Use imagery which appeals to all five senses, since many people have a
greater sensitivity to some senses than to others, e.g. setting sail in boat: see
ripples, smell and taste salt tang, feel wind, hear waves slapping against
boat, etc. Then land on island and see what it is like.

(c) Identifications

These are visualisations in which you 'become' something or somebody else
and identify with the feelings you imagine they might have.

330. Plant

Imagine you are a plant/tree/rosebush . . . where are you growing? . . . how
big? . . . what sort of flowers and fruits? . . . feel your roots . . . and your
branches . . . what is your life like? . . . how does it change with the seasons?
. . . what do you feel about it? . . . what are the surroundings like? . . . are
you on your own? . . . what can you see? Afterwards, paint your plant and
its environment, and talk about it in the first person, as it was in the
visualisation.

331. Natural Objects

Visualisations of self as tree, flower, house, etc. A flower is a good one to
start with, as for most people this is an image without negative meanings.

332. Dialogues

Dialogues between some of these, e.g. visualisations of self as a treestump,
then a cabin, then a stream, followed by dialogues between any of these.

333. Moving Objects

Visualisations of self as a moving object, such as an animal or motorbike.

334. River

Image of a river – imagine being the source of a stream (source) . . . which tumbles down (childhood) . . . into a bold and powerful river (youth) . . . becomes a larger river, polluted and carrying cargo (responsibility) . . . then to an estuary . . . and finally the sea (loss of ego).

335. Mythical Character

Imagine being a mythical character . . . setting out on a journey . . . where to? . . . having adventures . . . what sort of adventures? . . . finally arrive home again. After the journey do a painting about the journey or one aspect of it.

(d) Other ways of stimulating imagery

336. Group Fantasy

Heads in a circle, one person starts with what she/he sees in imagination, then another takes over, creating group fantasy.

337. Relaxation, Meditation and Painting

This is a method used by Dorothy Cameron (1996) with homeless people. People come to the group and do an immediate first painting about how they are feeling, to let off steam. This is followed by a period of relaxation and meditation, sometimes with music, sometimes with guided imagery. Then group members do a second, more reflective, painting in a calmer state of mind. Discussion includes both paintings.

Further reading

Cameron, D. (1996) 'Conflict resolution through art with homeless people', in M. Liebmann (ed.) *Arts Approaches to Conflict*, London: Jessica Kingsley Publishers.

338. Listening to Music

Use music to create atmosphere, for example:

- Ravel: *Daphnis and Chloe*
- Brahms: *Symphony No. 1 in C (3rd Movement)*
- Respighi: *The Pines of Rome*
- Debussy: *Girl with the Flaxen Hair*

Or any other music with pleasant-feeling possibilities.

339. Breathing in Light

Can be a good way to end a session

Breathe deeply . . . be aware of the group as a circle . . . imagine glow of light round each person . . . gradually watch light join into complete circle . . . notice how far light spreads out . . . follow it gently . . . imagine breathing in this light . . . going down into chest . . . spreading into body . . . name each part . . . and out through fingers and toes . . . feel the light and warmth . . . come back to familiar self and open eyes.

(e) Visualising change

340. Personal Development

Visualise yourself doing something you have always wanted to do, then do a picture about an aspect of what you saw.

Variation: visualise yourself overcoming a problem or dealing with it in a new way.

341. Saying Goodbye

Go into a garden . . . seated on the ground or a bench is someone you have lost . . . you greet each other and talk a while . . . there is something you would like to have said to that person before you lost them . . . this is an opportunity to say it . . . soon after your conversation comes to an end . . . you say goodbye . . . you both leave the garden, but in opposite directions. When you come out of the visualisation, paint any aspect of it that was particularly meaningful.

Variation: paint or make an object to commemorate your taking leave.

(f) Further reading

Below is a list of books on guided imagery and visualisation:

Guided imagery and visualisation

Achterberg, J., Dossey, B. and Kolkmeier, L. (1994) *Rituals of Healing: Using Imagery for Health and Wellness*, New York: Bantam Books.
Gawain, S. (2002) *Creative Visualization*, Novato, CA: New World Library.
Gawler, I. (1998) *The Creative Power of Imagery: A Practical Guide to the Workings of Your Mind*, London: Deep Books.
Leuner, H. (1984) *Guided Affective Imagery: Mental Imagery in Short-Term Psychotherapy, the Basic Course*, New York: Thieme Medical Publications.

Levine, S. (2000) *Guided Meditations, Explorations and Healings*, Basingstoke: Gill and Macmillan.

Mason, L. J. (2001) *Guide to Stress Reduction*, Berkeley, CA: Celestial Arts.

Samuels, M. (1988) *Seeing with the Mind's Eye: The History, Techniques and Uses of Visualization*, New York: Random House.

Stevens, J. O. (1989) *Awareness: Exploring, Experimenting, Experiencing*, London: Eden Grove.

Guided imagery and music

Bonny, H.L. and Summer, L. (2002) *Music and Consciousness: The Evolution of Guided Imagery and Music*, Gilsum, NH: Barcelona Publishers.

Bruscia, K. and Grocke, D. (2002) *Guided Imagery and Music: The Bonny Method and Beyond*, Gilsum, NH: Barcelona Publishers.

2. DREAMS, MYTHS AND FAIRY TALES

342. Working with Dreams

Paint a dream or nightmare you have had, especially one that is important or recurrent, or most recent. Variations:

(a) If dreams are not remembered, paint a daydream or fantasy.
(b) Use Gestalt technique (see p. 49) on images in dream painting, to explore them in the present tense.
(c) With an unhappy dream, create (visually or verbally) a more satisfactory ending.
(d) Keep a journal of dreams and thoughts arising, in words or pictures.
(e) Write a poem about the dream or painting of it (the abbreviated forms of blank verse poetry lend themselves to expressing dream images).
(f) Start with a key 'snapshot' of a particular moment in the dream, then do an image of the scene before and the scene after.

343. Daydreams and Fantasies

Make up a fantasy story in six small pictures, or specify the kind of story: adventure, day you would like, etc. Variations:

(a) Close eyes and look inside – paint what you see.
(b) Paint any fantasy or daydream you have.
(c) Deal with people you know in a series of fantasy drawings.
(d) Paint your New Year's resolutions.
(e) Select from various landscape photographs and create a fantasy about your place.

344. Clay Monsters

Create a 3-D monster from fantasy or dreams.

345. Stories and Strip Cartoons

Draw out a page into boxes and make up a story of any kind (useful way to start if timid). Variations:

(a) Changing a picture into something different in three moves.
(b) Strip cartoons.

346. Myths

Write or paint the story of your life as a myth. Variations:

(a) Imagine stepping into a parallel world, the Essential Myth of yourself, of which your everyday self is only a small part. Paint your myth.
(b) Draw identifications with personal heroes and villains, and act them in a play.

347. Fairy Tales

Using a traditional fairy tale as a starting point, read aloud. Then everyone does a painting, open ended or on a specified aspect, and meets to discuss. Variations:

(a) Ask people to change the ending, or stop before the end and ask people to supply their own ending, or imagine the next scene.
(b) Use any sort of story in the same way.

3. PAINTING AS MEDITATION

348. Meditative Drawing and Painting

Close eyes, relax and concentrate on bodily sensations. Stay with body awareness until you have clear images, then draw abstractly to communicate experience. Variations:

(a) Concentrate on a sound, word or syllable.
(b) Meditate or focus on a particular object, an apple, a stone, etc., in its entirety, and make brush marks to express feelings.
(c) (Zen technique) Imagine becoming the essence of the selected object. Draw during or after.

(d) Hold some clay and mould it for a few minutes as a centring activity.
(e) Use clay as reflective medium after an intense experience.
(f) Make clay pinchpot and stay centred so pot becomes balanced.

Many more possibilities are given in the following workbook: Cook, C. and Heales, B. C. (2001) *Seeding the Spirit: The Appleseed Workbook*, Birmingham: Woodbrooke Quaker Study Centre, 1046 Bristol Road, Birmingham BS29 6LJ. Tel: 0121 472 5171. email: enquiries@woodbrooke.org.uk. Website: www.woodbrooke.org.uk.

349. Mandala Possibilities

A mandala is a balanced, centred design, in which opposites are integrated. Mandalas are found in illustrations of Eastern mythology and Jung paid great attention to them. It is often a good idea to start a session on mandalas with some sort of relaxation or meditation, to become aware of a centre for the mandala, and of the opposites to work with. Some ideas for mandala possibilities:

(a) Your day and your night, and the transitions from one to the other.
(b) The present year, or your lifespan.
(c) Your body, top and bottom, right and left, front and back.
(d) Inner and outer experience; thinking and feeling; masculine and feminine.
(e) Mandala with different sections for aspects of your life.
(f) Make a mandala with another person, exploring differences and relationships.
(g) Mandala of balanced colours.
(h) Mandalas using stories of gardens, e.g. Garden of Eden, story of Buddha, etc.

Further reading

Dahlke, R. (1992) *Mandalas of the World: A Meditating and Painting Guide*, New York: Sterling.
Fincher, S. (1991) *Creating Mandalas: for Insight, Healing and Self-Expression*, Boston: Shambhala.
Jung, C. (1983) *Man and His Symbols*, London: Picador.

350. Autogenic Training

This is a progressive relaxation technique which can be done using art therapy methods as well as the more conventional verbal methods. It is useful for dealing with chronic problems, physical and mental.

(a) Relaxation exercise: after body relaxation, paint with watercolour brush in leisurely way, broad horizontal bands of colour with varying tones of greens, blues and purples, being aware of paint spreading across the page. Continue until in relaxed state.
(b) Visualisation: with eyes closed, visualise a pleasant experience, and verbalise it. Then paint your visualisation.
(c) Make another painting or clay model of how you felt during your trip.
(d) Paint or sculpt your problem, and compare with any work on this theme before the relaxation.

Further reading

Landgarten, H. (1999) *Clinical Art Therapy*, New York: Brunner/Mazel.
Mason, L. J. (2001) *Guide to Stress Reduction*, Berkeley, CA: Celestial Arts.

351. Colour Meditations

These are done on wet paper using watercolour paints and soft brushes. Thoroughly wet the paper (cartridge or watercolour paper) and smooth down onto flat board (plywood is good), easing out air bubbles from the centre with a sponge. Then apply one particular colour and watch what happens. The process of doing colour washes can be treated as a relaxation or meditation. Combinations of different colours can evoke different feelings and give rise to definite forms which 'grow' out of the painting. Variations:

(a) Paint with eyes closed.
(b) Paint with two brushes, one in each hand, with a different colour on each brush.

Wet paper painting has been developed particularly by members of the Anthroposophical Movement based on the work of Rudolf Steiner. Further details from the Rudolf Steiner Bookshop (tel: 020 7724 7699) or the library (tel: 020 7224 8398) at Rudolph Steiner House, 35 Park Road, London NW1 6XT. Information also from Wellspring Bookshop (Rudolf Steiner Book Trust), 5 New Oxford Street, London WC1A 1BA (tel: 020 7405 6101).

Further reading

Collot d'Herbois, L. (2000) *Light, Darkness and Colour in Painting Therapy*, Edinburgh: Floris Books.
Hauschka, M. (1985) *Fundamentals of Artistic Therapy*, London: Rudolf Steiner Press.

Mayer, G. (1983) *The Mystery Wisdom of Colour*, London: Mercury Arts.
Mees-Christeller, E. (1985) *The Practice of Artistic Therapy*, Spring Valley, NY: Mercury Press.

K   Links with other arts

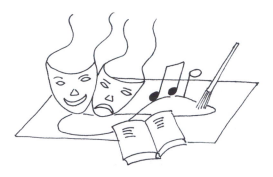

Visual art is often used in conjunction with movement, drama, poetry and music. The ideas in this section are those which specifically combine visual art with another mode of expression. There is an infinite number of ways of combining the different arts, and those given below are only a few of the possibilities. Those wanting to develop this area should consult the growing literature in these fields. There is also a list of arts therapy organisations in the Resources section at the end of this book. This section looks at visual art combined with the following other arts:

- Movement
- Drama
- Words and poetry
- Sound and music
- Multi-media.

Movement

352. Trust Walks

In pairs, lead each other on a blind walk, introducing partner to as many textures as possible. Come back and paint the experience. Variations:

(a) Paint the experience of being the leader or of being led.
(b) Paint as a group on a large sheet of paper.
(c) Do breathing exercises, then draw how you feel afterwards.
(d) Touch hands and faces of others (eyes closed). Remember any images passing through your mind. Write or draw these afterwards.

353. Emotions

Use movement to explore and express emotions, then paint the experience, for example:

(a) Meeting as friends and as enemies.
(b) The sea: group forms a circle and expresses moods of ocean waves, calm, storm, etc.
(c) Move to music.

354. Gesture Drawings

Make marks on paper with a gesture communicating an inner feeling. These can be developed into a larger picture. Variations:

(a) Make marks on separate pieces of paper and play a guessing game with others as to which was which.
(b) Choose pairs of opposites, e.g. anger and calm, joy and despair, etc.
(c) Try with left and right hands.
(d) Imagine hand is a bird swooping, ant crawling, bulldozer, etc. and change colour each time. Move to new sheet of paper when full. Choose ways you like best and least and contemplate differences.
(e) See also no. 270(b) – movements of different qualities.
(f) Make vigorous movements to describe stance and rhythm of an object and repeat them until you can 'feel' the object. Then record these feelings on a large piece of paper.
(g) Close eyes, draw pattern in the air with hand and develop into a rhythm. Then transfer it to paper and give it a title.
(h) As in (g), but start by imagining a good feeling.

355. Acting Sensations

Imagine moving through peanut butter, or syrup, etc. Act it and then paint the sensation.

356. Dance

After dancing as a group, paint feelings on large piece of paper.

Drama

357. Sculpting Situations

Each person draws a diagram of how she/he feels about the group, prefer-ably abstract. Each person's diagram is then used to create a human sculpture from the group. The person who did the drawing alters the sculpture if not correct. Variations:

(a) Let the sculptures 'come alive' and see what happens.
(b) Make models from clay or plasticine, then act situations using the models. This can be done at many levels.
(c) See also Family Sculptures – nos. 190 and 213.
(d) See also no. 268 – Group Roles, and no. 269 – Role Playing.

358. Dialogues

Use contrasts or conflicts which arise from a painting or model to develop a dialogue, e.g. between a hard and soft aspect of self. Invent voices for each part. After a dialogue, try to see if there is a 'middle way' combining both qualities.

359. Action and Conflict Themes

Combine painting and drama around any suitable themes, for example:

(a) No. 123, Action and Conflict Themes.
(b) No. 309, Situation Diagrams.
(c) No. 315, Trading Skills.
(d) Themes from other sections.

360. Elements and Conflict

Divide group members (or they choose themselves) into roughly equal numbers of the four elements. Ask each group to devise a short piece of drama/movement to demonstrate to the others. This can then develop into improvised drama/movement together. Then ask them to contribute to a group painting in their different styles. Discussion can pick out conflicts and complementary aspects of these styles.

   Variation: ask each group to look at the positive and negative qualities of their element and how to communicate with the other elements. Group painting can look at how groups can co-exist peacefully.

361. Accidents

Act dramas of accidents and injuries, involving the use of plaster of Paris gauze for sculptures, plaster casts, etc. Good for children. Variations:

(a) Use plasticine models to rehearse impending difficult situations, operations, hospital stays, etc.
(b) Re-enact any situations which have recently caused distress.
(c) Role reversal, in which children have control. e.g. giving injections, etc.

362. Pictures Come to Life

Everyone draws a picture on a theme connected with their present situation. Then they make their pictures come alive and enact the situation. Variations:

(a) Develop drama to include any changes people want to make in themselves or their situation.
(b) Pictures of the future and enact them.
(c) Use drama tableaux based on pictures.
(d) Bring dreams to life and enact different endings.

363. Masks

(a) Make masks and use them in improvisations and plays. See also nos. 134, 232, 281.
(b) Monster masks: make 'scary monster' masks and use them to act plays and situations. (This can be a useful way of approaching situations involving anger, especially for younger groups.) Sometimes a useful counterpart to this is also to make 'happy monster' masks.
(c) Make masks to develop different fantasy 'cultures'. Add customs and observable behaviour and act out the cultures. Bring two cultures together to see how they interact.

364. Hats

Each person makes a different hat and wears it. Then the group works out a drama to include the different personalities represented.

365. Drama Games

Almost any drama game or 'warm-up' can be followed by painting. This gives a chance for reflecting on an experience, although it is not always possible to 'translate' directly from one mode to another. For co-operative games, see the Resources section at the end of book. For drama games, contact the British Association for Dramatherapists, address in Resources section.

366. Puppet Theatre

Make puppets and use them in improvisations and plays. There are many kinds of puppets, e.g. glove and finger puppets, string puppets, shadow puppets, full-size puppets. A variety of materials can be used, e.g. cloth, papier-mâché (see no. 74), junk materials, paperbags, etc. In addition, drawings can be made at any stage, related to the story, the characters or the puppets.

367. Theatrical Costumes

Draw yourself in theatrical costume (everyday and fantasy). Develop the role and use it in a group improvisation.

368. Storytelling and Plays

A variety of other activities can be used to stimulate storytelling and play acting:

(a) Sand play (see no. 71).
(b) Paper figures (see nos. 60(e), 198(b)).
(c) Imaginary traffic system (see no. 89).
(d) Add images to a group painting, telling the story as it proceeds (see no. 250).
(e) Elements and conflict (see no. 360).
(f) Celebrating diversity (see nos. 133, 259)
(g) Masks (see nos. 134, 232, 281, 363).
(h) Puppets (see no. 366).
(i) Some other themes from previous sections which lend themselves to dialogues and plays:

- C: no. 83
- D: nos. 113, 119, 121, 122, 123
- E: nos. 127, 135, 140, 148, 155, 157, 165, 167, 171
- F: nos. 189, 190, 195, 196, 210, 213
- G: nos. 227, 238, 239
- H: nos. 249, 252, 258, 260, 262, 269
- I: nos. 276, 278, 314, 315
- J: nos. 342, 346

369. Tape Recorder

Use a tape recorder to describe paintings afterwards, or make associations with particular images (some people find tape recorders very inhibiting, others find them very liberating).

Variation: in pairs, interview each other about artwork done.

Words and poetry

370. Words to Image

Ask group members to call out words and write them on a piece of paper or card, or pass round a piece of paper for people to write down words. These words build up into associations and can then be used as a starting point for pictures.

Variation: cut out unrelated words from magazines. Then add images and put them together in any appropriate way.

371. Story Consequences Explored

Start with a round of 'consequences' in which everyone writes a sentence, passes it to the next person, who adds a sentence and folds over the previous sentence. Only the last sentence is showing each time the paper is passed on. At the end, members of the group read out the stories, generally amidst laughter. Usually issues are also brought up which can then be explored through painting or other arts.

372. Poetry as Stimulus

Use poetry read aloud as a stimulus for painting. Evocative poetry open to many interpretations works best, e.g. 'Ode to Autumn' (Keats), 'The Prophet' (Khalil Gibran), nonsense poems such as 'Jabberwocky' (Lewis Carroll), etc. Variations:

(a) Poetry reading as an activity in its own right.
(b) Responding to poetry with more poetry.
(c) Extend to collections of inspirational phrases.
(d) Use and make up Japanese haiku (short poems with three lines of blank verse) to provide starting points for pictures. There are some examples in Connell, C. (1998) *Something Understood: Art Therapy in Cancer Care*, London: Wrexham Publications.

373. Poetry as Response

As a change from painting, individuals can respond in poetry or word form to a group experience. This is particularly useful when the group has produced a painting telling a group story (see no. 249).

374. Concrete Poetry

This gives visual shape to words and combines words into an image; e.g. a poem about a fish in the shape of a fish; words placed in such a way as to express their meaning.

375. Journals

Many people keep diaries and can be encouraged to keep a diary or journal of their progress and feelings about the group. These journals can include drawings, collage and poetry as well as prose.

Sound and music

376. Sounds into Paint

Sit in a circle and make the same sound for 30 seconds, all together. Then walk about briskly, making all sorts of odd sounds. Next, stand back to back in the centre and make a silly sound. Finally, go to your own place at the edge of the room, put your hands over your ears and listen for your own inner sound. Start making it, continuing as you take your hands off your ears and become aware of others. Total time for this is about two minutes. Then do a painting of whatever occurs. Variations:

(a) With eyes closed, make a sound and draw to it for ten minutes, then open eyes and elaborate design.
(b) Play sounds from a variety of instruments, then paint in response to each sound.
(c) As above but use clay.

377. Name Sounds

Dramatically enunciate own name, with body movement to match. Identify other members by sound and gesture, and draw these.

378. Moulding Sounds

Use clay to mould into shapes appropriate to particular sounds, preferably with eyes closed.

379. Painting to Music

Paint to music in any way that it moves you. This can be done as an individual or as a group. Music which has a range of moods and is not too well known is most suitable. Some suggestions:

Classical

Bach; Beethoven symphonies; Berlioz: *Symphonie Fantastique*; Dvorak: *Piano Concerto*; Mahler symphonies; Vivaldi: *Concerto for Two Guitars*.

Contemporary

Kronos Quartet; Steve Reich.

Jazz

Keith Jarrett (piano works); Miles Davis: *Kind of Blue*; Jan Garbarek (saxophone).

World Music

Nasrat Fateh Ali Khan; Ravi Shankar; Tibetan bells; Andean pipes; African music; other types of traditional music.
  Variations:

(a) Listen to the music first, then play again and paint to it.
(b) Listen to the music several times and paint images evoked afterwards.
(c) Paint to the music quickly, using a succession of sheets of paper.
(d) Compare reactions to music, preferences, feelings evoked, images, etc.
(e) Some good music for children: *Peter and the Wolf*, *Swan Lake*, etc.
(f) See also no. 270.
(g) Select three short pieces of music (with the most intense one in the middle, calmer ones at beginning and end) and ask group members to respond in images after each piece of music.
(h) Group painting to music.
(i) Use music that reminds you of different seasons.
(j) Paint to music for exercises that bring together group contributions, see no. 242, 264.

See also Resources section for books on Guided Imagery and Music, and the address of the Association for Music and Imagery.

380. Life Chart to Music

After drawing a lifeline or life chart (see no. 140), sit in front of it and compose a series of sounds to complement your story.

Multi-media

381. Letters

Make letters of the alphabet using dancing, music and painting. Good for children.

382. Evocative Adjectives

Choose an evocative adjective, and express it in several different modes, e.g. percussion, words, movement, paint.

383. Scents

Use different scents as a stimulus to drawing and painting.

384. Stimulus to Paint

Use any medium – music, poetry, short story, movement, dance, etc. – to stimulate feelings which can be painted.

385. Response to Paint

Respond to paintings in terms of poetry, song, movement, etc.

386. Sensory Awareness

This exercise aims to improve awareness of the environment and draw attention to sensory experience. This is 'Denner's Technique', which is based on the theory that emotional tensions block perception (Denner 1967). Objects are provided to look at, smell, listen to and touch. Then rhythms, curves and other impressions are transferred to huge sheets of paper on the wall or floor and are continued into a free-flowing drawing. Variations:

(a) Lie down, eyes closed, explore world around using' smell, touch, hearing. Then move about, contacting objects and people. Open eyes and draw picture of world experienced.

(b) Use all five sense to examine objects, colours, shapes, sounds, and see what feelings are evoked. Find an appropriate means of expression for these.

387. Music and Movement

Move to music in the way it suggests, or according to a particular theme. Then paint this experience. See below and comments under no. 379 concerning suitable music:

(a) Compression and expression: Erik Satie's piano music.
(b) Cocoon: Debussy's *Reverie*.
(c) Gravity: Tchaikovsky's *Dance of the Sugar Plum Fairy*.
(d) Exploring possibilities: African drumming.
(e) Dancer: Borodin's *In the Steppes of Central Asia*.
(f) Growing: Erik Satie's or Chopin's piano music.
(g) Evolution: Gabr Szabo's piano music.
(h) Separation and connection: Aaron Copland's *Clarinet Concerto*.

388. Series of Sessions

Plan or evolve a series of sessions involving use of different arts media, as seems appropriate, e.g. movement to music, mural painting, drama, dance, poetry, relaxation, etc. This can be structured around a common theme or evolve from week to week. (See, for instance, Jennings and Minde 1994.)

389. Multi-media Events

Plan events and sessions round a theme (e.g. no. 258, Solidarity), using painting, music, poetry, drama, etc.

References

Denner, A. (1967) *L'Expression plastique, pathologie, et rééducation des schizophrènes*, Paris: Editions Sociales Françaises.

Jennings, S. and Minde, A. (1994) *Art Therapy and Dramatherapy: Masks of the Soul*, London: Jessica Kingsley Publishers.

L Media cross-reference

This section simply indicates by number the themes and exercises that mention particular media. Many others can, of course, be adapted for use with a desired medium.

1 **Pencils**

2 **Crayons**　　　almost all the ideas in this book

3 **Paint**

4 **Collage**
  - B. Media Exploration: nos. 42, 43, 60, 61, 62, 66, 69
  - C. Concentration, Dexterity and Memory: nos. 79, 80, 82, 90, 91, 92, 93, 95, 98, 99, 101, 102
  - D. General Themes: nos. 109, 116, 118, 119
  - E. Self-perceptions: nos. 125, 127, 128, 129, 132, 133, 134, 135, 140, 142, 143, 144, 145, 148, 159, 162, 172, 175, 176
  - F. Family Relationships: nos. 188, 197, 211
  - G. Working in Pairs: nos. 224, 230, 232, 236
  - H. Group Paintings: nos. 259, 260, 261, 262, 264, 267
  - I. Group Interactive Exercises: nos. 277, 293, 297, 304, 314, 316
  - J. Guided Imagery, Dreams and Meditations: nos. 343, 370

5 **Clay**
  - B. Media Exploration: nos. 70, 72, 75, 76
  - D. General Themes: nos. 116, 121
  - E. Self-perceptions: nos. 126, 127, 131, 132, 137, 154, 156, 157, 162, 172
  - F. Family Relationships: nos. 188, 190, 194, 198, 213
  - G. Working in Pairs: nos. 225, 234, 236
  - H. Group Paintings: nos. 251, 254, 260, 266, 268
  - I. Group Interactive Exercises: no. 272

- J. Guided Imagery, Dreams and Meditations: nos. 344, 348, 350
- K. Links with Other Arts: nos. 357, 361, 376, 378

6 Other 3-D and junk materials
- B. Media Exploration: nos. 43, 55, 60, 61, 65, 66, 67, 68, 69, 71, 72, 73, 74, 77, 78
- C. Concentration, Dexterity and Memory: nos. 83, 89, 103, 106
- D. General Themes: nos. 107, 113, 114, 116, 119
- E. Self-perceptions: nos. 125, 126, 127, 128, 131, 137, 141, 143, 147, 148, 151, 152, 153, 154, 155, 166, 167
- F. Family Relationships: nos. 190, 194, 198, 213, 214, 215
- G. Working in Pairs: no. 236
- H. Group Paintings: nos. 251, 254, 260, 263, 264, 266, 268
- I. Group Interactive Exercises: nos. 275, 276, 281, 282, 284, 302, 310, 313, 315
- J. Links with Other Arts: nos. 357, 359, 361, 364, 366, 368

7 Masks
- B. Media Exploration: no. 74
- E. Self-perceptions: nos. 127, 134, 152, 153, 154, 162, 184, 185
- G. Working in Pairs: nos. 232, 233
- I. Group Games: nos. 281, 288
- K. Links with Other Arts: nos. 363, 368

M   Media notes

This section includes a few very brief notes on different media and their particular advantages. Only the most readily available media are included here. For a list of catalogues of art materials, see Resources section at the end of the book.

1   Dry media
2   Paints
3   Brushes and other painting implements
4   Paper
5   3-D materials
6   Collage materials
7   Adhesives
8   Folders

Dry media

Pencils, crayons, felt-tip markers, etc. These are easier to control than wet or fluid media. This can be important for those with disabilities which make the mechanics of using fluid media difficult. They can also be useful for people starting off, if they are afraid to use paints and need to retain control over their medium to feel safe. On a practical level, many situations allow only dry media, e.g. home visits with materials, rooms which have to be kept clean or have no access to water, sessions which are too short to allow time to set out or clear up, and so on.

Pencils

The easiest to control, but difficult to get a strong effect or blocks of colour. Good quality ones can be expensive. For ordinary pencils, soft ones (2B, 3B, 4B) are easier to use than hard pencils. Erasers and pencil sharpeners are also needed. Pencil sharpeners of different sizes may be needed.

Watercolour pencils

These can be used as pencils in the usual way, but can also be dipped in water to use as watercolour paints.

Fibre/felt-tip pens and markers

Easy to use, good clear colours. Strong effects possible, but expanses of colour difficult. Good quality ones can be expensive. Thick markers are good for making a quick impact.

Wax crayons

Moderately easy to control, do not wear down quickly, cheap, large sizes available. Sometimes difficult to get good depth of colour. Good for children. Also useful for people who need to press really hard. Some adults find them difficult because of the associations with childhood. As well as the traditional colours, wax crayons are now available in metallic colours (bronze, silver and gold), which are popular with children and adults.

Oil pastels

Moderately easy to control, strong colours, variety of textures and blocks of colour possible. Reasonably priced.

Chalks and pastels

Moderately easy to use, but effects can smudge easily and need fixing. Chalks are cheap, but difficult to get a great range of colours. Artists' pastels contain toxic pigments. Some clients really enjoy the range of textures that can be achieved. Good range of colours usually available.

Charcoal

Quite difficult to use, smudges easily, but very good for strong effects and large drawings.

Graphite sticks

Same purpose as charcoal, but not as smudgy or breakable.

Skin-tone colours

Some dry media are available in skin tones of different shades and colours, e.g. wax crayons. This is important in our multicultural society.

Paints

Paints are much more fluid and therefore more difficult to control than dry media, but also much more rewarding in the effects that can be obtained, and more enjoyable to use for many people. Many artists' quality paints are toxic, so it is better to use scholastic materials. The paints below are all used with water.

Watercolours

The most fluid and difficult to control, mistakes cannot be corrected. This can be daunting, but can also help people to accept their mistakes and live with them. Available in tubes and in sets of little blocks – tubes are often easier to use. Moderately expensive.

Powder paint

Cheap, but difficult to achieve the desired consistency, and can be messy to use unless pre-mixed. Not very easy to use thickly or to correct mistakes.

Ready-mixed paint

These are the same paint as powder colour, but mixed ready to use. Thick, easy to use, reasonably cheap. Available in large plastic bottles. Can achieve strong effects. Changes tone as it dries, to less vibrant colours. Nozzles often clog up – useful to have a large paperclip on hand to unblock. As well as the traditional colours, they are now available in fluorescent colours (popular with children and adolescents) and metallic colours – bronze, silver and gold (popular with everyone). These are all more expensive than ordinary colours.

Acrylic and polymer paints

Easy to use, variety of textures possible. Paints dry very quickly, mistakes are easy to correct. Can achieve strong effects. Expensive. When dry, not soluble in water, so care needed with brushes.

Fingerpaints

Thick, good tactile quality, good for messy and regression work, and for children. Expensive.

Palettes

These are needed to put out and mix paints. Sturdy plastic ones with six or nine wells are best, but old plates and discarded small plastic trays can be used.

Water containers

These can be glass jars, plastic pots, etc. Containers should have a stable base. For young children there are non-spill plastic pots with tightly fitting lids.

Brushes and other painting implements

It is important to have a good range of sizes, especially larger ones:

- *hog, bristle, nylon*: range of sizes up to size 12, for general use, round and square
- *sable, ox hair or squirrel hair*: a few fine brushes for detailed work
- *house decorating brushes*: for large-scale work
- *sponges on sticks*: interesting alternative to brushes
- *sponges*: for spreading paint and for making prints
- *rollers*: different widths and materials (sponge, rubber) for large paintings
- *junk materials to paint with*: variety of these for different effects
- *adaptations (if needed)*: use holders, bandages or plastic balls for extra grips.

Paper

This can be an expensive item, but it is worth trying to ensure that a range of sizes is available, including large size. A range of colours is good too (including black), but if money is limited, white, grey or buff will suit most purposes. Paper should be thick enough to be enjoyable to use.

Sugar paper

Reasonably cheap, good for most paints, charcoal and pastels.

Cartridge paper

Good for watercolour paints and drawing. Quite expensive. Available in different weights.

Newsprint

Thin and cheap. Can sometimes obtain ends of roll from newspaper offices, stationery firms or 'Scrapstore' schemes. Gives large-size paper.

Lining paper

Cheap. Comes in rolls from decorating suppliers, so needs cutting to size. Rather narrow. Tears easily.

Card

Useful for heavy paint and collages using junk and natural materials. Can be expensive, but offcuts are often obtainable from scrapstores and resource centres.

3-D materials

Malleable 3-D media are good for themes involving strong feelings, especially anger, because people can use some of the energy associated with the feelings to work the media.

Plasticine and clayola

Easy to use, not messy, easily portable, fairly cheap. Good for children. Some adults find its associations with childhood difficult. Not easy to use for large-scale work or for very fine work.

Playdough

Good for children. Cheap, easy to make and use (see no. 75 for recipes).

Fun stuff

Easier to mould than plasticine and does not dry out. Available in fluorescent colours.

Fimo

Useful for fine work and can be baked in an ordinary oven to harden. Wide range of colours, including fluorescent and metallic. Expensive.

Clay

Messy, not easily portable, needs firing in a kiln if work is to be kept. Despite these difficulties, working with clay has many more possibilities than plasticine and is a completely different experience in feel and texture. Also good for letting off steam and large-scale projects. Reasonably cheap.

Nylon-reinforced clay

Does not need firing, can be painted or varnished when dry, but texture not as good as ordinary clay. Also more expensive. Useful in places where no kiln is available.

Junk materials

Variety of textures and methods of fixing available, large-scale projects possible. Good for expending energy if tools are used such as saw, hammer and nails.

Mask materials

Plaster of Paris bandages (available from chemists), paper bags, or pre-formed blank masks (available cheaply in bulk from most of the big catalogues for art materials – see Resources section). Masks can also be made from stiff paper, card, paper plates or papier-mâché over clay or a blown-up balloon (which is later popped).

Other materials

- Plaster of Paris in powder form. Big tubs usually available from catalogues. Fairly cheap. Messy to use and need to work fast before it sets. Useful for large projects.
- Polyfilla – useful for slower working as it does not set so fast, but more expensive.
- Pipecleaners – useful for small 3-D work. Reasonably cheap.
- Straws – good for blowing paint.

See also Section B – Media Exploration.

Collage materials

Magazines

Choosing images and arranging them can be a less daunting first step than actually making images, as it reduces anxiety about 'artistic performance'. It also has a 'distancing' effect in that the images chosen may, but do not have to, relate to the person who chose them. For instance, it may be easier to choose 'angry pictures' from magazines than to paint a picture of one's own anger. Difficult topics may sometimes be approached indirectly in this way. A wide variety of magazines is needed.

Travelling kits

A travelling kit of images can be useful to avoid carrying heavy magazines around. The collection needs to include a wide range of situations and people of all colours, cultures and types. Specialised collections can be made, e.g. people, landscapes, actions, etc.

Other collage materials

Other collage materials, such as fabrics, tissue paper, natural objects, junk materials, string, etc., can be used in addition to other media, or to explore textures and effects of different materials. Scrapstore schemes are available in many towns and cities.

   Glitter, sequins and other shiny materials are very popular, with adults as well as children.

Scissors

Good quality, sharp scissors are needed, but with rounded ends.

Adhesives

Glue sticks

These are easy to use, not messy, and easy to obtain in a variety of sizes. They are best for paper and light materials. They get used up very quickly.

Copydex

Rubbery emulsion, good for cloth.

Cow gum

Rubber solution, good for paper. Easy to peel off, so useful for shifting positions.

PVA

Water-based emulsion. When dry, not soluble in water. Good for paper, cloth, wood. Useful for collage and general purposes. Can also mix with powder or ready-mix paint to make plastic paint.

Glitter glue

This is a mixture of PVA-type glue and glitter, popular with children.

Polycell

Good for paper, papier-mâché, etc. Do not use heavy-duty variety containing fungicide.

Impact adhesive

Good for sticking wood and other materials quickly. But be careful of using glue which is flammable or has strong fumes.

Strong glue

There are other glues which stick wood and other materials more slowly than impact adhesives, such as Uhu, woodworkers' glue, etc. Avoid those which are flammable or have strong fumes.

Sticky tape

This includes clear or coloured Sellotape (single or double sided), brown parcel tape, masking tape and peel-off sticky labels. Parcel tape is strong but tricky to use. Masking tape is cheap, easy to use, can be peeled off and reapplied, and can be painted over – good for taping sheets together for a group painting.

Blu-Tak (or similar)

This is good for sticking things in temporary positions or fastening paper to walls, though it may take paint off walls when it is removed. If walls are precious, use it on doors. Can be reused.

Folders

Most groups need a way of storing members' pictures and other artwork. There is a variety of possibilities:

- home-made folders from large card and decorated by participants
- cardboard folders or clear wallets from one of the catalogues
- large clear portfolios with cardboard stiffening and 'plastic hole' handles
- large corrugated plastic portfolios with proper handles.

These go up in price according to quality.

List of contributors

Apologies to anyone whose name has been omitted. Putting together the second edition, as with the first one, has been very much a group effort.

Art therapists who took part in the survey in 1979

Cherry Ash
David Bostock
Caroline Case
Penny Campbell
Suzanne Charlton
Peter Cole
Paul Curtis
Michael Donnelly
Karen Lee Drucker
Michael Edwards
Douglas Gill
Andy Gilroy
Helen Greenwood
Julia Gudjonsson

Diana Halliday
Julie Hart
Roger Hart
Diana Hector
Robin Holtom
Pat Hurley
Tom Hutter
Sarah Kemp
Marion Kerswell
Adèle Lambert
Marian Liebmann
Maggie McKiernan
Gerry McNeilly
Jan Mallett

Patsy Nowell-Hall
Sue Parsons
Michael Pope
Meg Randall
Brian Richardson
Rita Simon
Claire Skailes
Roger Stanbridge
Jo Sutherland
Roy Thornton
Toril Valland Lowe
Roger Vickerman
Felicity Weir
Chris Wood

Further contributions in 1985

Sheena Anderson
Heather Buddery
Paul Curtis
Michael Donnelly
Karen Drucker

Jim Dymond
Tish Feilden
Helen Felton
John Ford
Sue Jennings

Linnea Lowes
Vicky Morrison
Tessa Roger-Jones
Beryl Tyzack

Art therapists who responded to a questionnaire for the second edition and contributed additional themes

Ann Bartholomew
Kate Broom
Jane Caven
Rebecca Conduit

Karen Drucker
Donella Kirkland
Sarah Lewis
Gemolyn McQuilkin

Georgina Rambton
Edy Scott
Budgie Summers
Sarah Tucker

Other contributions of themes to the second edition

Vicky Barber
Jupiter Daden
Judith Ducker
Jo Ferrell

Jane Habermehl
Herdeep Jassal-Wynter
Nicky Linfield
Diana van Loock

Richard Manners
Marian Miles
Nick Moore
Clare Sheridan

People who contributed to lists of books and organisations

Jenny Blayney
Bristol Cancer Help
   Centre
Leslie Bunt
Nadija Corcos
Anna Kälin

Cherry Lawrence
Mailout magazine
Helen Mason
Carla Paulo
Sarah Tucker
Diane Waller

Judy Weiser
Fiona Williams
Winford Manor
   Retreat Centre

Resources

The list of books and resources in this section is a selection of what is available, and is designed to give the reader further resources to pursue particular aspects. They are listed under the following headings:

1 Group work
2 Co-operative games and group activities
3 Art therapy with groups
   (a) Books focusing on art therapy with groups (general)
   (b) Books focusing on the use of themes in art therapy groups
   (c) Some art therapy books including chapters on groups
   (d) Family art therapy
   (e) Books used in compiling themes for the first edition of this book
4 Guided imagery and visualisation
5 Guided imagery and music
6 Mandalas
7 Anthroposophical approaches (Rudolf Steiner)
8 Recording
9 Evaluation and research
10 List of organisations
   (a) Art therapy organisations
   (b) Art materials
   (c) Other arts therapies organisations
   (d) Art and arts organisations
   (e) Evaluation and research
   (f) Other UK organisations
11 Journals and newsletters
   (a) Arts therapies
   (b) Participation in the arts

Those resources which have been consulted to gather themes are marked with an asterisk *.

1. Group work

Benson, J. F. (2001) *Working More Creatively with Groups*, 2nd edn, London: Routledge.

Brown, A. (1992) *Groupwork*, 3rd edn, Aldershot: Ashgate.

Douglas, T. (1991) *A Handbook of Common Groupwork Problems*, London: Tavistock/Routledge.

Dwivedi, K. N. (ed.) (1993) *Group Work with Children and Adolescents: A Handbook*, London: Jessica Kingsley Publishers.

Phillips, J. (2001) *Groupwork in Social Care: Planning and Setting Up Groups*, London: Jessica Kingsley Publishers.

Sharry, J. (2001) *Solution-Focused Groupwork*, London: Sage.

Whitaker, D. S. (2001) *Using Groups to Help People*, 2nd edn, Hove: Brunner-Routledge.

Yalom, I. D. (1995) *The Theory and Practice of Group Psychotherapy*, 4th edn, New York: Basic Books.

2. Co-operative games and group activities

Bond, T. (1986) *Games for Social and Life Skills*, London: Hutchinson.

Luvmour, S. and Luvmour, J. (2002) *Win–Win Games for All Ages: Cooperative Activities for Building Social Skills*, Gabriola Island, BC: New Society Publishers. (Distributed in UK by Jon Carpenter Publishing, Charlbury, Oxon.)

Masheder, M. (1991) *Let's Play Together: Cooperative Games for All Ages*, London: Green Print.

Orlick, T. (1982) *The Second Cooperative Sports and Games Book*, New York: Random House. (Published in UK by Writers' and Readers' Cooperative 1983.)

Woodcraft Folk (1996) *Games, Games, Games II*, 2nd edn, London: Woodcraft Folk. (Available from Woodcraft Folk, 13 Ritherdon Road, London SW17 8QE.)

3. Art therapy with groups

(a) Books focusing on art therapy with groups (general)

Riley, S. (2001) *Group Process Made Visible: Group Art Therapy*, Hove: Brunner-Routledge.*

Skaife, S. and Huet, V. (eds) (1998) *Art Psychotherapy Groups: Between Pictures and Words*, London: Routledge.

Waller, D. (1993) *Group Interactive Art Therapy: Its Use in Training and Treatment*, London: Routledge.*

(b) Books focusing on the use of themes in art therapy groups

Barber, V. (2002) *Explore Yourself Through Art: Creative Projects to Promote Personal Insight, Growth and Problem-solving*, London: Carroll & Brown.*

Campbell, J. (1993) *Creative Art in Groupwork*, Bicester: Speechmark (formerly published by Winslow Press).*

Jennings, S. and Minde, A. (1994) *Art Therapy and Dramatherapy: Masks of the Soul*, London: Jessica Kingsley Publishers.

Liebmann, M. F. (1996) *Arts Approaches to Conflict*, London: Jessica Kingsley Publishers.*

Liebmann, M. F. (2003) *Art Therapy for Groups*, 2nd edn, Hove: Brunner-Routledge.

Luzzatto, P. (2000) 'The creative journey: a model for short-term group art therapy with posttreatment cancer patients', *Art Therapy: Journal of the American Art Therapy Association*, 17, 4: 265–9.*

Makin, S. R. (1999) *Therapeutic Art Directives: Activities and Initiatives for Individuals and Groups*, London: Jessica Kingsley Publishers.*

Robbins, A. (1994) *A Multi-Modal Approach to Creative Art Therapy*, London: Jessica Kingsley Publishers.*

Ross, C. (1997) *Something to Draw On: Activities and Interventions using an Art Therapy Approach*, London: Jessica Kingsley Publishers.*

Safran, D. S. (2002) *Art Therapy and AD/HD: Diagnostic and Therapeutic Approaches*, London: Jessica Kingsley Publishers.*

Silverstone, L. (1997) *Art Therapy: The Person-Centred Way*, 2nd edn, London: Jessica Kingsley Publishers.

(c) Some art therapy books including chapters on groups

Adamson, E. (1984) *Art as Healing*, London: Coventure.

Betensky, M. G. (1995) *What Do You See? Phenomenology of Therapeutic Art Expression*, London: Jessica Kingsley Publishers.

Campbell, J., Liebmann, M., Brooks, F., Jones, J. and Ward, C. (eds) (1999) *Art Therapy, Race and Culture*, London: Jessica Kingsley Publishers.

Case, C. and Dalley, T. (1990) *Working with Children in Art Therapy*, London: Tavistock/Routledge.

Case, C. and Dalley, T. (1992) *The Handbook of Art Therapy*, London: Tavistock/Routledge.

Connell, C. (1998) *Something Understood: Art Therapy in Cancer Care*, London: Wrexham Publications.*

Dalley, T. (ed.) (1984) *Art as Therapy: An Introduction to the Use of Art as a Therapeutic Technique*, London: Tavistock.

Dalley, T., Case, C., Schaverien, J., Weir, F., Halliday, D., Nowell Hall, P. and Waller, D. (1987) *Images of Art Therapy: New Developments in Theory and Practice*, London: Tavistock.

Dokter, D. (ed.) (1994) *Arts Therapies and Clients with Eating Disorders: Fragile Board*, London: Jessica Kingsley Publishers.

Dokter, D. (ed.) (1998) *Arts Therapists, Refugees and Migrants: Reaching Across Borders*, London: Jessica Kingsley Publishers.

Gilroy, A. and Dalley, T. (eds) (1989) *Pictures at an Exhibition*, London: Tavistock/Routledge.

Gilroy, A. and McNeilly, G. (eds) (2000) *The Changing Shape of Art Therapy*, London: Jessica Kingsley Publishers.

Hagood, M. (2000) *The Use of Art in Counselling Child and Adult Survivors of Sexual Abuse*, London: Jessica Kingsley Publishers.*

Hiscox, A. R. and Calisch, A. C. (eds) (1998) *Tapestry of Cultural Issues in Art Therapy*, London: Jessica Kingsley Publishers.

Hogan, S. (ed.) (1997) *Feminist Approaches to Art Therapy*, London: Routledge.

Hogan, S. (ed.) (2003) *Gender Issues in Art Therapy*, London: Jessica Kingsley Publishers.

Kalmanowitz, D. and Lloyd, B. (1997) *The Portable Studio: Art Therapy and Political Conflict: Initiatives in Former Yugoslavia and South Africa*, London: Health Education Authority.

Kalmanowitz, D. and Lloyd, B. (eds) (in press) *Art Therapy and Political Violence*, Hove: Brunner-Routledge.

Killick, K. and Schaverien, J. (eds) (1997) *Art, Psychotherapy and Psychosis*, London: Routledge.

Liebmann, M. (ed.) (1990) *Art Therapy in Practice*, London: Jessica Kingsley Publishers.*

Liebmann, M. (ed.) (1994) *Art Therapy with Offenders*, London: Jessica Kingsley Publishers.

Malchiodi, C. A. (ed.) (2002) *Handbook of Art Therapy*, New York: Guilford Press.

Moon, C. H. (2001) *Studio Art Therapy: Cultivating the Artist Identity in the Art Therapist*, London: Jessica Kingsley Publishers.

Murphy, J. (ed.) (2000) *Art Therapy with Young Survivors of Sexual Abuse: Lost for Words*, Hove: Brunner-Routledge.

Rees, M. (ed.) (1998) *Drawing on Difference: Art Therapy with People who have Learning Difficulties*, London: Routledge.

Riley, S. (1999) *Contemporary Art Therapy with Adolescents*, London: Jessica Kingsley Publishers.*

Sandle, D. (ed.) (1998) *Development and Diversity: New Applications in Art Therapy*, New York: Free Association Books.

Waller, D. and Gilroy, A. (eds) (1992) *Art Therapy: A Handbook*, Buckingham: Open University Press.

(d) Family art therapy

Arrington, D. B. (2001) *Home Is Where the Art Is: An Art Therapy Approach to Family Therapy*, Springfield, IL: C.C. Thomas.

Kwiatkowska, H. (1978) *Family Therapy and Evaluation Through Art*, Springfield, IL: C.C. Thomas.

Landgarten, H. (1987) *Family Art Psychotherapy: A Clinical Guide and Casebook*, New York: Brunner/Mazel.

Linesch, D. (1997) *Art Therapy with Families in Crisis: Overcoming Resistance Through Nonverbal Expression*, New York: Brunner/Mazel.

Linesch, D. (2000) *Celebrating Family Milestones: By Making Art Together*, Toronto: Firefly Books.

Proulx, L. (2003) *Strengthening Emotional Ties through Parent–Child-Dyad Art Therapy*, London: Jessica Kingsley Publishers.

Wadeson, H. (1980) *Art Psychotherapy*, Chichester: John Wiley.

(e) Books used in compiling themes for the first edition of this book

Cortazzi, D. and Roote, S. (1975) *Illuminative Incident Analysis*, New York: McGraw-Hill.*

Denner, A. (1967) *L'Expression plastique, pathologie, et rééducation des schizophrènes*, Paris: Editions Sociales Françaises.*

Donnelly, M. (1983) 'The origins of pictorial narrative and its potential in adult psychiatry', unpublished research diploma thesis, Department of Art Therapy, Gloucester Rouse, Southmead Hospital, Bristol.*

Harris, J. and Joseph, C. (1973) *Murals of the Mind*, New York: International Universities Press.*

Keyes, M. F. (1974) *The Inward Journey*, Millbrae, CA: Celestial Arts.*

Kwiatkowska, H. (1978) *Family Art Therapy*, Springfield, IL: C. C. Thomas.*

Landgarten, H. B. (1981) *Clinical Art Therapy*, New York: Brunner/Mazel.*

Liebmann, M. F. (1979) 'A study of structured art therapy groups', unpublished MA thesis, Birmingham Polytechnic.*

Luthe, W. (1976) *Creativity Mobilisation Technique*, New York: Grune and Stratton.*

Oaklander, V. (1978) *Windows to Our Children*, Moab, UT: Real People Press.*

Pavey, D. (1979) *Art-Based Games*, London: Methuen.*

Rhyne, J. (1996) *The Gestalt Art Experience: Patterns that Connect*, Chicago: Magnolia Street Publishers.*

Robbins, A. and Sibley, L. B. (1976) *Creative Art Therapy*, New York: Brunner/Mazel.*

Rubin, J. A. (1978) *Child Art Therapy*, New York: Van Nostrand Reinhold.*

Ulman, E. and Dachinger, P. (eds) (1976) *Art Therapy in Theory and Practice*, New York: Schocken.*

Ulman, E. and Levy, C. A. (eds) (1980) *Art Therapy Viewpoints*, New York: Schocken.*

Wadeson, H. (1980) *Art Psychotherapy*, Chichester: John Wiley.*

4. Guided imagery and visualisation

Achterberg, J., Dossey, B. and Kolkmeier, L. (1994) *Rituals of Healing: Using Imagery for Health and Wellness*, New York: Bantam Books.

Cook, C. and Heales, B. C. (2001) *Seeding the Spirit: The Appleseed Workbook*, Birmingham: Woodbrooke Quaker Study Centre.

Gawain, S. (2002) *Creative Visualization*, Novato, CA: New World Library.

Gawler, I. (1998) *The Creative Power of Imagery: A Practical Guide to the Workings of Your Mind*, London: Deep Books.

Leuner, H. (1984) *Guided Affective Imagery: Mental Imagery in Short-Term Psychotherapy, The Basic Course*, New York: Thieme Medical Publications.

Levine, S. (2000) *Guided Meditations, Explorations and Healings*, Basingstoke: Gill and Macmillan.

Mason, L. J. (2001) *Guide to Stress Reduction*, Berkeley, CA: Celestial Arts.

Samuels, M. (1988) *Seeing with the Mind's Eye: The History, Techniques and Uses of Visualization*, New York: Random House.

Stevens, J. O. (1989) *Awareness: Exploring, Experimenting, Experiencing*, London: Eden Grove.*

5. Guided imagery and music

Bonny, H. L. and Summer, L. (2002) *Music and Consciousness: The Evolution of Guided Imagery and Music*, Gilsum, NH: Barcelona Publishers.
Bruscia, K. and Grocke, D. (2002) *Guided Imagery and Music: The Bonny Method and Beyond*, Gilsum, NH: Barcelona Publishers.

6. Mandalas

Dahlke, R. (1992) *Mandalas of the World: A Meditating and Painting Guide*, New York: Sterling Publishing.
Fincher, S. (1991) *Creating Mandalas: For Insight, Healing and Self-Expression*, Boston: Shambhala.
Jung, C. (1983) *Man and His Symbols*, London: Picador.

7. Anthroposophical approaches (Rudolf Steiner)

Collot d'Herbois, L. (2000) *Light, Darkness and Colour in Painting Therapy*, Edinburgh: Floris Books.
Hauschka, M. (1985) *Fundamentals of Artistic Therapy*, London: Rudolf Steiner Press.
Mayer, G. (1983) *The Mystery Wisdom of Colour*, London: Mercury Arts.
Mees-Christeller, E. (1985) *The Practice of Artistic Therapy*, Spring Valley, NY: Mercury Press.

Further details from the Rudolf Steiner Bookshop (tel: 020 7724 7699) or the library (tel: 020 7224 8398) at Rudolph Steiner House, 35 Park Road, London NW1 6XT. Information also from Wellspring Bookshop (Rudolf Steiner Book Trust), 5 New Oxford Street, London WC1A 1BA (tel: 020 7405 6101).

8. Recording

Case, C. and Dalley, T. (1992) *The Handbook of Art Therapy*, London: Tavistock/ Routledge.
Whitaker, D. S. (2001) *Using Groups to Help People*, 2nd edn, Hove: Brunner-Routledge.

It is worth consulting books on groupwork for a range of methods of recording and evaluation.

9. Evaluation and research

American Art Therapy Association (1992) *A Guide to Conducting Art Therapy Research*, Mundelein, IL: American Art Therapy Association. Website: <www.arttherapy.org>

CORE & OQ details. See list of organisations in section 10(e), p. 336.

Department of Health (2001) *Treatment Choice in Psychological Therapies and Counselling: Evidence Based Clinical Practice Guidelines*, London: NHS Executive. Website: <www.doh.gov.uk/mentalhealth/treatmentguideline/index.htm>

Duncan, B. and Miller, S. (2000) *The Heroic Client: Doing Client-Directed, Outcome-Informed Therapy*, San Francisco: Jossey-Bass.

Gantt, L. and Tabone, C. (1998) *Formal Elements Art Therapy Scale Manual*, West Virginia: Gargoyle Press.

Gilroy, A. (2003) *Art Therapy, Research and Evidence Based Practice*, London: Sage.

Gilroy, A. and Lee, C. (eds) (1995) *Art and Music: Therapy and Research*, London: Routledge.

Kalmanowitz, D. and Lloyd, B. (1997) *The Portable Studio: Art Therapy and Political Conflict: Initiatives in former Yugoslavia and South Africa*, London: Health Education Authority.

McDowell, I. and Newell, C. (1996) *Measuring Health: Guide to Rating Scales and Questionnaires*, 2nd edn, Oxford: Oxford University Press.

McNiff, S. (1998) *Art-Based Research*, London: Jessica Kingsley Publishers.

National Health Service (1999) *National Service Framework for Mental Health*, London: Department of Health. Website: <www.doh.gov.uk/nsf/mentalhealth.htm>

National Health Service (1999) *Clinical Governance: Quality in the New NHS*, London: NHS Executive. Website: <www.doh.gov.uk/clinicalgovernance>

National Health Service (2001) *Information for Research Governance*, London: Department of Health. Website: <www.researchinformation.nhs.uk/main/governance.htm>

Ogles, B. M., Lambert, M. J. and Field, S. A. (2002) *Essentials of Outcome Measurement*, New York: Wiley.

Parry, G. and Watts, F. N. (eds) (1996) *Behavioural and Mental Health Research: A Handbook of Skills and Methods*, Hove: Psychology Press.

Payne, H. (ed.) (1993) *Handbook of Inquiry in the Arts Therapies: One River, Many Currents*, London: Jessica Kingsley Publishers.

Roth, A. and Fonagy, P. (1996) *What Works for Whom? A Critical Review of Psychotherapy Research*, New York: Guilford Press.

Rowland, N. and Goss, S. (eds) (2000) *Evidence-Based Counselling and Psychological Therapies: Research and Applications*, Hove: Routledge.

Sharry, J. (2001) *Solution-Focused Groupwork*, London: Sage.

10. List of organisations

(a) Art therapy organisations

Australia

Australian National Art Therapy Association (ANATA)
PO Box 303 Glebe
NSW 2037
Australia
E-mail: annette.coulter@bigpond.com (sec)
Australia-wide tel: 1300 557 002

Canada

The art therapy associations in Canada are mostly regional.

British Columbia Art Therapy Association
Website: www.arttherapy.bc.ca

Canadian Art Therapy Association (CATA)
26 Earl Grey Road
Toronto ON
M4J 3L2
Canada
Tel: (416) 461 9420
Website: www.catainfo.ca

Ontario Art Therapy Association
Website: www.oata.ca

Quebec Art Therapy Association
Website: www.iquebec.ifrance.com/aatq/english7.html

UK

British Association of Art Therapists
The Chancery Room
16–19 Southampton Place
London WC1A 2AJ
Tel: 020 7745 7262
Fax: 020 7745 7101
E-mail: baat@gateway.net
Website: www.baat.org

Studio Upstairs
Diorama Arts Centre
34 Osnaburgh Street
London NW1 3ND
Tel: 020 7916 5431
Fax: 020 7916 5477
E-mail: mail@studioup.u-net.com
Website: www.diorama-arts.org.uk

USA

American Art Therapy Association
1202 Allanson Road
Mundelein
Illinois 60060-3808
USA
Tel: +1 847 949 6064
Fax: +1 847 566 4580
E-mail: info@arttherapy.org
Website: www.arttherapy.org

International

International Networking Group of Art Therapists (ING/AT)
Contact: Gaelynn P. Wolf Bordonaro, Membership Coordinator &
Newsletter Editor
PO Box 4125
Louisville KY 40204-4125
E-mail: gaelynn@hotmail.com
Nancy Slater, Key Networker: slaterna@esumail.emporia.edu
Hannah Sherebrin, Book Review Editor: sherebri@actcom.co.il

(b) Art materials

Scrapstores and resource centres

The following website lists the Scrapstores and Resource Centres (which
recycle industrial off-cuts to schools and social projects) in the UK:

Website: www.geocities.com/rainforest/wetlands/4936/index.htm
E-mail: www.scrapstores@btinternet.com

Art and craft catalogues (for materials)

Consortium – Tel: 0845 330 7770. Website: www.theconsortium.co.uk
Galt – Tel: 0870 242 4477. Website: www.galt-educational.co.uk
Great Art – Tel: 0845 601 5772. Website: www.greatart.co.uk
Hope Education – Tel: 0161 366 2900. Website: www.hope-education.co.uk
NES Arnold – Tel: 0845 120 4525. Website: www.nesarnold.co.uk
Nottingham Rehab – Tel: 0845 120 4522. Website: www.nrs-uk.co.uk
Specialist Crafts Art Design – Tel: 0116 269 7711. Website: www.speccrafts.co.uk
Step by Step – Tel: 0845 125 2550. Website: www.sbs.educational.co.uk

(c) Other arts therapies organisations

Association for Dance Movement Therapy (UK)
c/o Quaker Meeting House
Wedmore Vale
Bristol BS3 5HX
E-mail: query@admt.org.uk
Website: www.admt.org.uk

British Association for Dramatherapists
41 Broomhouse Lane
Hurlingham
London SW6 3DP
Tel/fax: 020 7731 0160
E-mail: gillian@badth.demon.co.uk
Website: www.badth.co.uk

Association of Professional Music Therapists
61 Churchill Road
East Barnet
Herts EN4 8SY
Tel/fax: 020 8440 4153
E-mail: apmtoffice@aol.com
Website: www.apmt.org.uk

British Society for Music Therapy
61 Churchill Road
East Barnet
Herts EN4 8SY
Tel: 020 8441 6226
Fax: 020 8441 4118
E-mail: info@bsmt.org
Website: www.bsmt.org

European Consortium for Arts Therapies Education (ECArTE)
c/o Christine Lapoujade, Chair
Universite René Descartes Paris
Centre de Formation Continue
45 rue des Saints
Peres
75006 Paris IV
France
Tel: 0033 142 862 291
Fax: 0033 142 862 159
E-mail: sylviane.frederic@cfc.univ-paris5.fr
Website: www.uni-muenster.de/Ecarte/index.html

International Expressive Arts Therapies Association
PO Box 320399
San Francisco
CA 94132-0399
USA
Tel: (415) 522-8959
E-mail: webmaster@ieata.org
Website: www.ieata.org

South African Network for the Arts Therapies Organisations (SANATO)

Western Cape

Angela Rackstraw
22 Alpina Rd
Claremont 7708
Western Cape
South Africa
Tel/fax: +27+21 683 9654
E-mail: angrack@mweb.co.za

Gauteng

Mercedes Pavlicevic
c/o Music Therapy Programme
Dept of Music
University of Pretoria
Pretoria 0002
South Africa
Tel: +27+12 420 5372
Fax: +27+12 420 4517
E-mail: mercedes@postino.up.ac.za

Virtual Arts Therapies Network
University of Derby
School of Education, Health and Science
Mickleover Campus
Derby DE3 5GX
Tel: 01332 592149
Fax: 01332 514323
E-mail: s.hogan@derby.ac.uk
Website: www.derby.ac.uk/v-art/

(d) Art and arts organisations

Association for Music and Imagery
PO Box 4286
Blaine WA 98231-4286
USA
Tel: (360) 756-8096
Fax: (360) 756-8097
E-mail: ami@nas.com
Website: www.bonnymethod.com/ami

In the UK, contact:

The MusicSpace Trust
St Matthias Campus (UWE)
Oldbury Court Road
Fishponds
Bristol BS16 2JP
Tel: 0117 344 4541
Fax: 0117 344 4542
E-mail: musicspace@uwe.ac.uk

Conquest Art Centre
(art for physically disabled people)
Cox Lane Day Centre
Cox Lane
West Ewell
Surrey KT19 9PL
Tel/fax: 020 8397 6157
Website: www.conquestart.org

Creative Exchange
(creative activity in sustainable development)
Business Office 1
East London Centre
Boardman House
64 Broadway
Stratford
London E15 1NT
Tel: 020 8432 0550/1
Fax: 020 8432 0559
E-mail: info@creativexchange.org
Website: www.creativexchange.org

Koestler Award Trust
(annual exhibition of art made in prisons)
9 Birchmead Avenue
Pinner
Middlesex HA5 2BG
Tel: 020 8868 4044
Fax: 020 7261 1263
E-mail: dsalmon@koestler.freeserve.co.uk
Website: www.hmprisonservice.gov.uk/life/

National Network for the Arts in Health
123 Westminster Bridge Road
London SE1 7HR
Tel: 020 7261 1317
Fax: 020 7261 1263
E-mail: info@nnah.org.uk
Website: www.nnah.org.uk

Unit for the Arts and Offenders
Neville House
90–91 Northgate
Canterbury
Kent CT1 1BA
Tel: 01227 470629
Fax: 01227 379704
E-mail: info@a4offenders.org.uk
Website: www.a4offenders.org.uk

(e) Evaluation and research

Art Therapy Practice Research Network (ATPRN)
Contact: Val Huet and Neil Springham
23 St James
London SE14 6NW
Tel: 020 7919 7171 ext 4046
E-mail: ATPRN@gold.ac.uk

CORE IMS
Contact: John Mellor-Clark
47 Windsor Street
Rugby CV21 3NZ
Tel: 01788 546019
Fax: 01788 331407
E-mail: admin@coreims.co.uk
Website: www.coreims.co.uk

OQ-45 (Outcome Questionnaire)
Website: www.oqfamily.com/
See also Ogles, B.M., Lambert, M.J. and Field, S.A. (2002) *Essentials of Outcome Measurement*, New York: Wiley.

UK Clearing House on Health Outcomes at the Nuffield Institute for Health
71–75 Clarendon Road
Leeds LS2 9PL
Tel: 0113 233 3940
Fax: 0113 246 0899
E-mail: hsschho@leeds.ac.uk
Website: www.leeds.ac.uk/nuffield/infoservices/UKCH/home.html

(f) Other UK organisations

Commission for Racial Equality
St Dunstan's House
201–211 Borough High Street
London SE1 1GZ
Tel: 020 7939 0000
Fax: 020 7939 0001
E-mail: info@cre.gov.uk
Website: www.cre.gov.uk

DIAL (Disability Information Advice Line) UK
St Catherines
Tickhill Road
Doncaster DN4 8QM
Tel: 01302 310123
Fax: 01302 310404
E-mail: dialuk@aol.com
Website: www.dialuk.org.uk

Disability Rights Commission
DRC Helpline
FREEPOST
MID 02164
Stratford upon Avon
CV37 9BR
Tel: 08457 622 633
Textphone: 08457 622 644
Fax: 08457 778 878
E-mail: enquiry@drc-gb.org
Website: www.drc-gb.org

Health Professions Council
Park House
184 Kennington Park Road
London SE11 4BU
Tel: 020 7582 0866
Fax: 020 7820 9684
E-mail: info@hpc-uk.org
Website: www.hpc-uk.org

11. Journals and magazines

(a) Arts therapies

Arts in Psychotherapy. Published by Elsevier Science in New York and Amsterdam. (USA) email: usinfo-f@elsevier.com. (Europe, Middle East and Africa) email: nlinfo@elsevier.com. Websites: www.elsevier.com/homepage and www.elsevier.nl/locate/artspsycho

Art Therapy: Journal of the American Art Therapy Association and *AATA Newsletter*. Both from American Art Therapy Association, details above.

AT Newsbriefing (newsletter of British Association of Art Therapists), c/o BAAT (address above).

Inscape (journal of British Association of Art Therapists), c/o BAAT (address above).

International Arts Therapies Journal (online), see Virtual Arts Therapies Network for contact details. Website: www.derby.ac.uk/v-art/journal/

International Networking Group of Art Therapists' Newsletter. Editor: Gaelynn P. Wolf Bordonaro. E-mail: gaelynn@hotmail.com. Book Review Editor: Hannah Sherebrin. E-mail: sherebri@actcom.co.il

Theoretical Advances of Art Therapy. Bi-annual British conference, with information and abstracts on website: www.taoat.org.

(b) Participation in the arts

The Bulletin. Published by the Unit for the Arts and Offenders (address above).

Conquest Art Magazine. Published by Conquest Art Centre (address above).

Creative Exchange Bulletin. Published by Creative Exchange (address above).

Mailout (national magazine for developing participation in the arts) 87 New Square, Chesterfield, Derbyshire S40 1AH, E-mail: info@e-mailout.org, Website: www. e-mailout.org

Index

Note: Capitalised entries refer to organisations, authors and art therapists, and titles of practical exercises